Sugar

Sugar

A TALE OF MOTHERHOOD & MEDICINE

Raissa Hacohen

ISBN-13: 9781518816246
ISBN-10: 151881624X
Library of Congress Control Number: 2016900282
CreateSpace Independent Publishing Platform
North Charleston, South Carolina

Prelude

To my dearest son,

I hope you cannot recall these childhood memories, but I will never forget them. They will sit idle in my mind, seeping and spilling over into my thoughts and emotions when I wake and when I sleep. The path to and through parenthood is by far the most challenging and trying time I have ever experienced.

I wrote this so that when we rejoice together, our joy will be that much sweeter knowing what we have overcome as a family. I wrote this so that one day, when these challenges have been long overcome, you will know the depth of our love and gratitude for health, for each other, and for you. I wrote this so that when you are a teenager and the apathy of adolescence is burning inside you, you can remember that once upon a time, I tried really, really hard.

I began writing this journal for me. In the darkest of times, the pen and paper (so to speak) were my only solace. I continued to write it for you so that you would know your story, our story, and how much we have overcome so that anything else we face will shrink in comparison.

We decided to publish this journal for others, with the hope that other parents and children, other partners and families, can find strength in our journey. If this helps even one person get through one more hour of one more day, we will consider it worthwhile. We remember the times that flew by and the times that inched minute by minute. We remember the highs of your first smile, first word, first step, and the lows of your hospitalization, diagnosis, and treatment.

We are privileged to be your parents. To call you our son. To see you get better day by day. To say good-bye to your medications and medical equipment bit by bit. We still have a long way to go, but we see it now—the light at the end of the tunnel. And we remember the days that were all darkness and despair.

We dedicate this book to those who are currently experiencing the darkness. To those who are enveloped by it. To those who can't imagine a life before or after it. We were you once. Continue to hope. Continue to dream. Just *continue.* Get out of bed in the morning. Put one foot in front of the other. Like the ants, continue to march. Just doing that makes you a very brave person.

And remember, be kind. For everyone you meet is fighting a harder battle.

—Mother Teresa

CHAPTER 1

Hope

I WISH FOR YOU
Your father's height and his kind eyes.
I hope you have his patience and his diplomacy.
I hope that things come with enough ease that you avoid frustration and worry
And that things are challenging enough that you understand their full worth—
The most rewarding things always come with a little sweat and a few tears.
I hope you know how truly special you are,
How many miles were traveled and oceans crossed in order for your story to begin.
And I hope you know how much you are loved and how blessed we feel to be your family.

I wrote this for you on April 28, 2013. I was four months pregnant with you, and I felt you kick for the first time. So teeny tiny, almost imperceptible. I was in corpse pose, resting at the end of my prenatal yoga class, which I attended twice a week until another five months and fifty pounds slowed my physical capabilities and my will to be anywhere but floating in a pool of water.

Those were the good days, full of hope and endless possibility.

CHAPTER 2

In the Beginning

YOUR FATHER AND I MET on a hike in the desert. I was a senior in college, on winter break in Israel, and an Israeli friend of mine from Brown invited me to go hiking with his friends in Wadi Kelt, a riverbed that meanders through the desert. Your father was tall and handsome, with kind eyes and a smile that drew you in. He called to ask me out the next day and took me to a restaurant on Usishkin Street, one that no longer exists. Then we walked around town and sipped hot cocoa from Babette, a French waffle bar, the richest hot chocolate in town. We walked to the Old City of Jerusalem and scaled a locked gate to climb the Old City walls.

Scaling walls with thousands of years of history—and there we were beginning ours. It would be on these walls over the old Zion Gate where your father would propose to me, where we would celebrate our anniversaries. All in the dark of night, under the glow of the moon, in a clandestine spot on the Old City walls. Our spot. Sitting on thousands of years of history while making our own.

Women have a small window during their lifetimes in which they are endowed with superpowers—the ability to incubate and carry life inside their own bodies. The power to give birth, produce milk, and nourish a life. Five years into our marriage, I too was endowed with superpowers—and there you were, a teeny-tiny dot on a big ultrasound screen. You were but a gentle heartbeat, and we were so excited to meet you. We called you Tulip those first few months, as you were but a tiny bud waiting to flower. Our job was to water you.

CHAPTER 3

Calm before the Storm

IT WAS A RELATIVELY QUIET pregnancy, aside from the one time that we rushed to the emergency clinic for internal bleeding.

One morning, I woke up with a little bit of blood and panicked. I woke up your *abba*, sobbing hysterically. I thought I'd lost you then. I was inconsolable.

We rushed to the emergency clinic. And when the doctor found you, safe and sound, beating gently, I thanked God for saving you and promised that if I were lucky enough to be a mother, at the end of this long journey, I would do everything I could to protect you.

Little did I understand how insignificant my power and ability would be and how many millions and billions of things—large and small—would have to go right in order for me to fulfill that promise.

CHAPTER 4

The Birth

NINE MONTHS AND FIFTY POUNDS later, I was so eager to meet you. I enjoyed having you inside me, kicking my tummy to wake me up every morning. *Thump, thump, thump!* I started calling you Kung Fu Panda.

It was week thirty-eight with Rosh Hashanah fast approaching. The Jewish New Year was two weeks before my due date, but your grandmother (Safta) wanted to fly in. She had a premonition that you would come early.

We hosted a big family dinner on the evening of Rosh Hashanah, and even as I was hosting, I noticed that you were less vocal. I felt less movement and less kicking. I thought it was odd, but I figured that you were just sleeping. Then the next morning, you didn't wake me up with kicks, and my concern started to mount. Where were you? What were you doing? So we grabbed the hospital bag and decided to go to the hospital to get checked. Better safe than sorry.

The roads were completely empty. Total quiet. The silence was deafening, the same way the roads are quiet after a big snowstorm in New England, where I grew up. Yet here in the Middle East, there are no snowstorms, just the quiet of the New Year holiday. With people spending time with their families, we sped to the hospital without another car in sight.

We arrived at the hospital, and the staff admitted me as a patient. Took our vitals. Did an ultrasound. They located your heartbeat and assured us that you were OK, but you still weren't moving. So they monitored us for hours on end. Still no movement. They stuffed me with sugars in order to wake you up. I have never eaten so much junk food in my whole life. They had me force tea, candy, Snickers, and challah with honey down my throat. They continued to monitor, but still nothing.

Concern started to escalate. The doctor on call said that they were discussing whether to induce me with the possibility of a C-section or whether to send me straight to the operating room. They decided on an emergency C-section. They notified us five minutes before sending me to the operating room.

A nurse started prepping me, and Safta came in to give me a hug and wish me luck, but the tears in her eyes and quiver in her voice gave her away. She was terrified. Scared in a way only a parent can be. Afraid to lose you. Afraid to lose me. Afraid because once you are rolled into surgery, you literally have no control—a feeling with which I was familiar and soon to be more intimately acquainted.

Your abba is the strongest man I know, and as he wheeled me through the operating room hallway in a wheelchair, I felt his feet drag. Even he gave away his mounting fear for you and for me as he kissed me on the forehead with tears streaming silently down his face. We said a prayer, asking God to protect us.

I don't remember much after that. The operating room was white and sterile. There must have been a staff of eight prepping me and the machines. Everyone looked busy and determined, each focused on his or her own tasks. I thought to myself that it seemed like a lot of people for just one surgery.

They put a blue sheet over my legs, and the anesthesiologist tapped my spine. The room started to blur. I don't remember anything beyond that, except feeling tension, a stretching kind of tension. As if they were stretching my body to each corner of the room. Incredible pulling. As if my body were a tent they were pitching. When you came out, I barely had enough strength to form the words, "Is my son OK?" And then it went dark.

CHAPTER 5

A Shell

I WOKE UP IN THE postop room. I use the term *woke up* loosely, since I think I just gained consciousness long enough to throw up. The room was pristine and white, with those terrible separator curtains that hospitals use to pretend you have some semblance of privacy.

The nurse came over and forcefully turned my head to the left so that I would vomit into this small liver-shaped piece of cardboard instead of choking on my own vomit. For that, I was grateful. It was a motion that I would become intimately familiar with over the next few days as I began to recover from a surgery that literally sliced me open from one side of my pelvis to the other, leaving behind a straight trail of staples, like breadcrumbs, as evidence of the event.

After a Cesarean section, you feel like Gumby. No control over your own limbs. To sit up, to move, to walk, you must learn again from scratch. I remember sitting on a plastic chair in the shower, staring at my feet. I couldn't reach them. It was too painful. I'd had months of not being able to see my feet during the pregnancy, and there I was, so close. I could see them, but I couldn't reach, certainly not well enough to wash them. As I let the water fall, I remember feeling humiliated. I had to call Mom to shower me, like when I was a child.

And while I was grateful to her for the assistance, I felt my self-esteem shrink, as I couldn't even perform regular daily tasks on my own. The physical pain was excruciating, but the emotional harm was worse. I remember feeling incredible guilt and humiliation that I wasn't strong enough, not womanly enough, to birth you properly. As I lay in bed, not strong enough to walk, not strong enough to move, I felt like a shell of my former self. This was not the strong-willed, healthy twenty-nine-year-old I knew. I was different, transformed. Transformed physically by surgery. Emotionally by motherhood. Little did I know that it would take me a long, long time to recover and again become the woman I once was.

The amount of guilt and shame that came along with that emergency C-section was overwhelming and unexpected. When we had taken our prenatal class, we'd had an entire session on C-sections. I knew it was an option, but I'd wished it away then, hoping that it was a card I wouldn't be forced to play. When Sareet, my friend and first visitor, came to the hospital, she could tell that I was holding on to a lot of anger and hurt surrounding the birth. My lack of control. My birth plans A, B, C, and D down the drain. My physical and emotional pain from the surgery.

She told me, "Raissa, you have to feel your feelings. Pushing them away to the back of your mind, ignoring them and fighting them, allows them to fester. Take a moment. Express them, feel your feelings, and *whoosh*, they'll fly away. Feel them in order to let them go."

And I did. I let the emotions of guilt, shame, and disappointment wash over me. And as quickly as I let them in, they disappeared—off to haunt someone else. To haunt someone else who was denying them.

CHAPTER 6

Freshman Orientation

The maternity ward is a weird parallel universe where mothers, young and old, are thrust together to recover from their respective birth experiences. Everyone is forced to stay two to five days for "observation," depending on how traumatic her birth was. C-section mothers are assigned to rooms together, as they need special observation and are compelled to stay longer.

The official patient attire was a hideous pink-patterned muumuu that had buttons strategically placed for easy breastfeeding access. All the healthy babies were kept together in the nursery for specific hours so that the mothers could sleep and recover. As far as nurses go, the maternity-ward nurses had the least power in the whole hospital. They patrolled the ward, taking temperatures and blood pressures and doling out Tylenol like candy.

I asked if they had anything stronger than Tylenol. They didn't.

You could tell the first-time mothers from the others, as we ended up wearing the muumuus the longest. Some women bounced back quickly and were already comfortable in their own clothes and skinny jeans just days after birth. Others (read: me) could spend weeks in those awful muumuus because, while hideous, they identified you as a patient, specifically a maternity patient, so everyone knew just by your outfit to excuse your physical appearance and to cut you a large amount of slack for being overtired and depressed, and for functioning at 3 percent of your normal mental capacity. You had just given birth, after all.

CHAPTER 7

Sophomore Orientation

While the maternity ward was its own universe that took some adjustment, the neonatal intensive care unit was its own galaxy, and we were clearly outsiders. While Safta nursed me back to health, your abba stayed vigilantly by your side. He sent me photos of you until I was mobile enough for Safta to wheel me over to the neonatal intensive care unit (NICU). Same floor, floor nine, but worlds away, considering I couldn't take three steps on my own.

As I was wheeled into the hallway, I saw photos lining the hall. Photos of healthy children who had spent time in the NICU, sent in by their grateful parents. Some were of twins, some with before and after photos, but all of perfectly healthy children, ipso facto.

As we passed the photos, my heart was full of sadness and hope that one day soon, we would also be able to send in a photo of our healthy son, and this experience would be all but a distant memory.

There is a big sign in red letters outside of the NICU that reads ENTRANCE PERMITTED ONLY FOR PARENTS AND GRANDPARENTS. ALL OTHER PERSONS AND FAMILY ARE FORBIDDEN. Of course, since Israelis are terrible at following rules, inevitably some families have three fathers, five grandmothers, and even children sneaking in to get a peek at their proud accomplishments. Often you would see parents holding up their babies and presenting them like Simba in the *Lion King* movie, while excited family members took photos from a distance at the entrance with their cell phones.

Because of the strict visiting rules, staff immediately identified visitors as "*Ima*," "*Abba*," "*Saba*," and "*Safta*," and that's how you were called for the rest of your stay. I was no longer Raissa, just Ima. And just like that, my place in the hierarchy of the hospital was identified. My disgusting pink muumuu gave me away, and I quickly became a fixture in the NICU, sitting vigilantly by your side—like all the other worried imas, hovering over the sixty other beds lining the NICU. We sat by our respective beds, poring over our children, tears streaming as we silently prayed to our respective gods for health, for strength, and for the day that we could take our babies home.

It was quickly apparent that the staff had its own hierarchy. There were the doctors, nurses, cleaning staff, and secretaries. Each group had its own internal hierarchy, too. The senior doctors, of which there were four, rotated monthly running the NICU. The residents were the young doctors each in charge of a number of babies—or as they called them, "patients"—and reported to the senior physicians. They were important because they were in charge of your baby's daily medical welfare, but impotent because they didn't have the authority to order or execute treatment without permission.

The nurses' hierarchy also stemmed from seniority. At the top of the chain were the middle-aged nurses, with thirty-plus years of experience in the NICU. These nurses got the best shifts—the morning shifts—and often the residents and even senior doctors would listen if they recommended a treatment. They were also the best nurses to get, because they took the best care of their babies. The younger nurses were kind but often less competent and less capable, more easily overwhelmed and more often fatigued, as they were forced to work the evening and late shifts. The cleaning staff—as cleaning and maintenance staff members often are—were invisible. They played a crucial but underappreciated role in the NICU, and no one seemed to notice or appreciate their contributions.

And the secretaries, as they often do, possessed a secret power that enabled them to access and order around the staff on all rungs of the ladders—doctors, nurses, and maintenance alike.

And, by the way, parents and grandparents fall way, way below, the lowest rung on the totem pole, even far below the maintenance staff. Yes, we, the parents, just created your patient, and yes, we played a vital role, but that is severely and immediately overlooked. Often parents were seen as obstacles in the patient's treatment—and they were certainly treated as such.

At first, since they didn't bother learning our names, we didn't bother learning theirs. We called each staff member according to his or her appearance or temperament, whichever was more pronounced. There was String Bean, a tall, stick-thin senior resident. There was Pompous, a senior physician who literally looked over or through everyone perceived to be below his level on the totem pole. There was Schlumpy, a senior doctor who was so unkempt that, outside of the NICU, he would have easily been mistaken for a homeless person, but who was the most agile, adept doctor in the whole unit at drawing blood and finding good veins on his teeny-tiny patients. There was also Grumpy, a senior nurse with an ostensible contempt for parents but a secret, gentle love that she showed toward her little patients. The list goes on. We had all the Seven Dwarfs, a series of emotions, and a handful of vegetable names for the NICU staff those first weeks.

The NICU is a sterile environment and must be kept that way for the health of the babies inside the unit. Visitors must sterilize their hands before entering and wear yellow or blue gowns that go over normal clothes. Initially, no one shared any of these rules with the parents, so most parents' first introduction into the NICU was taking three steps toward the door and having a nurse chase them out for wearing the wrong thing or failing to sterilize. I burst into tears the first time I was rolled into the NICU, when a nurse chased me out for failing to sterilize my hands. As I began to sob, I told her that I couldn't get up out of the wheelchair to reach the sink and wash my hands. Obviously, my outburst softened her a bit, and she brought over some hand sanitizer.

Mom then rolled me over to your station—or "giraffe," as they are called in the NICU. They're small, elevated rectangular beds with long necks supporting fluorescent white lights that heat the bed from overhead. And for the first time, I laid eyes on you, my little miracle.

CHAPTER 8

Ecstasy and Agony

MEETING YOU FOR THE FIRST time was, and is, the highlight of my life. I had imagined you, thought you into being, yearned to be your mother, carried you for nine months…and there you were. Instantly, all of my pain melted—the pain of being sliced like a loaf of bread, the humiliation and disappointment of not following my natural hypnobirthing plan, and the ache in my heart of not meeting you for the first few days of your life, of not being well enough to physically leave the maternity ward. It all dissipated with the excitement of seeing you for the first time, of getting to meet my little creation.

And as quickly as it dissipated, the pain came rushing back—intensified—in the form of motherhood. As I saw you lying on your tiny hospital bed, at the end of a row of beds designated for preemies, with other parents crying, sobbing, praying over their beds, arguing, negotiating, begging their respective deities for the health of their children, I was overcome with panic, fear, and worry.

You had your tiny little hand wrapped around your abba's finger, and he was cradling your head. It was all of you that we were allowed to touch, as you were hooked up to monitors: heart rate, breathing rate, and saturation. You had multiple IVs delivering a cocktail of drugs with names I couldn't pronounce, let alone remember. You had a tube stuck up your nose delivering continuous food and another tube across your face that pushed up your nostrils, helping deliver more oxygen into each breath you drew.

Although I was overwhelmed with all the medical equipment and beeping and lights and monitors, you were still the most beautiful creature I had ever laid eyes on. Hospital or no, you were my little boy, my pride and joy. And the first time you grabbed my finger, I was overcome with emotions. Joy for finally, finally, finally getting to meet you, and deep, deep, deep sorrow for the pain that you were experiencing in this horrible place called the NICU. Surely, I thought, we don't belong here. Surely we won't be here for long. Which, it turns out, is the lie all parents must tell themselves. The lie I told myself countless times during what would turn out to be a long, extended stay in the hospital.

We weren't allowed to pick you up, to hold you, to hug you, until you were six weeks old. One and a half months is a long, long time to wait to cradle your pride and joy. So in the meantime, we did all we could. We held your hand, cupped your head, and sang to you.

Honestly, I read every motherhood and baby book I could get my hands on to prepare, and none of them even remotely mentioned, let alone prepared me, for this type of situation. My mind was blank. In my post-surgery delirium, I forgot everything. Every song, every lyric I have ever known. All that came to me that day, and many of the days following it, was "The Ants Go Marching." And just like the ants, though paralyzed by fear and trepidation, I continued to march…praying that I would get to keep you.

CHAPTER 9

Seeking Answers

You were quickly diagnosed with hyperinsulinemia, a disease that means your pancreas produces too much insulin and causes low blood-sugar levels. It is the exact opposite of diabetes and generally a childhood disease. The doctors could not tell us whether it was permanent or transient, meaning it could disappear tomorrow or plague you into adolescence, which is quite a large gap for a parent to comprehend.

They initially identified the culprit for your condition as maternal diabetes during pregnancy—which, it turned out, I did not have. They began mapping our DNA to see if it was genetic and ran a hemoglobin A1C test to see if it was related to the pregnancy. So many questions and so few answers—some of which your medical team would discover, and many, many of which were simply beyond their power.

Unfortunately, that wasn't the only health issue you were contending with. You had a breathing tube, blood transfusions, a severe skin rash called fat necrosis (which looks like a serious case of frostbite across your back), liver failure, and a host of other health issues. You had a big heart defect, but you were too sick for it to be fixed. Off to a rocky start, and, to our dismay, we weren't taking you home any time soon. You and I were both still patients on the ninth floor, so abba packed up suitcases from the house, and we rented a room in a small in-house hostel on the fifth floor of the hospital. We didn't know it then, but room five would be our home for the next sixteen weeks. While four months doesn't sounds like a long time for a vacation or time off, it's a terribly, unbearably long time for a stay in the hospital.

Room five looked very much like the inside of a psychiatric ward. White, sterile walls. Minimal furniture made of fake wood. Two single beds, a closet, a desk. No windows, no fresh air. It crossed my mind a few times to decorate, but you could only book the room weekly. The reservation needed to be renewed every Sunday, and when Sunday rolled around, I could never bear the mental burden of planning to stay even one additional day, let alone another week in the hospital.

And this became my whole world, shuffling between the ninth and fifth floors. Abba, Safta, and I took turns watching over you. Waiting to be released from the prison that had just become our entire world. I felt conflicting emotions toward the hospital for keeping you alive and saving you while simultaneously locking you, our most prized possession, away.

CHAPTER 10

Depression

Those first few weeks in the hospital felt like an eternity. When I fell into my deepest, darkest despair, the words just came pouring out. The pen and paper became my only solace. God help me for letting some of these thoughts even cross my mind. I wrote:

Being a parent is hard.
You start building hopes and dreams
From the moment you hear that first heartbeat—
And then miraculously your life changes.
Instead of dreaming about which Ivy League (Brown, obviously)
And great loves and bigger adventures,
You are hoping for one good day. One hour of stable breathing. One more check with a stable sugar.
Praying for the day you get to introduce fresh air and unadulterated sunshine into your son's life. Waiting for the time you get to hold your son in the quiet of your own home. Just waiting. Waiting to live your real life. The one you imagined for your family. Outside the hospital walls. Waiting for the real beginning. Waiting to pretend that this was all just a bad dream. Waiting for the ruby slippers to appear. Waiting to utter, "There's no place like home. There's no place like home. There's no place like home." And suddenly you're home.

CHAPTER 11

Falling Deeper

How to lose your will to live:
You think it happens suddenly,
But in truth it happens slowly,
Like grating cheese,
And suddenly there is nothing left;
Your spirit is utterly broken,
Lying on the ground waiting to be resuscitated,
Praying to be reborn.

Nine weeks into our hospital stay, I went to yoga for the first time since giving birth. As I exited the hospital, climbed the hill up toward the gym, and crossed the train tracks, a thought crossed my mind, and I entertained it for ever-so-brief a moment. If I just put one foot out, just one step, perfectly timed as the train crossed the tracks, just dip my toe, this could all be over. This nightmare would be over. I could not endure any more suffering. Not for me, not for my family.

And as quickly as the thought entered my mind, I banished it to the furthest reaches of my soul.

After the train left the station, I continued on my way just in time to start sun salutations.

CHAPTER 12

A Patient Once More

My days were occupied with the intense stress and agonizing chronic depression of the NICU. Trying to be a good mother, good nurse, and good advocate in this environment was absolutely exhausting. No control and marginal input but maximum emotional, physical, and mental effort proved to be a draining combination.

One evening I spiked a fever—38.8 degrees Celsius, which is about 102 degrees Fahrenheit. We had lived in the hospital for the past few weeks, I had just returned my hospital gowns, and I couldn't bear to become a patient again. That stupid gown with an open back that left half your behind hanging out at all times and the horrible plastic wristband with your name and number that was impossible to remove. The IV permanently plugged into your arm that was constantly itchy and made you feel like a junkie. I just couldn't do it again.

I threw myself into an ice-cold shower and hopped back into bed. Sopping wet and shivering, I checked my temp again. One hundred and three. *Damn.* Time to walk the plank. Safta and Abba walked me down to the emergency room on the first floor, and I checked in for tests. They found my vein and inserted the IV tube, took my temperature, heart rate, blood pressure, and urine sample, and had me lie down in a bed.

As you start to feel yourself plunge into sickness, you start to let other things that would normally concern you fall by the wayside. Your hair, appearance, clothes, and smell all become irrelevant luxuries as the waves of illness overcome you.

The first course of action was to send me for a pelvic exam, as they suspected that my fever was a byproduct of the emergency C-section a few weeks prior. It showed nothing, so the doctor sent me to get a CT scan. CT scans are full-body scans in which you lie on a metal piece with your arms over your head as they insert you into a machine that scans your body. In order for the scan to read, you must first drink a disgusting material that tastes radioactive. I got through about half the necessary amount required before I puked all over the ER floor. I barely managed to choke down the other half before they gave me an injection and sent me into the scan.

As I lay down on the table and the technician altered my body position for optimal machine reading, I felt as if my veins were simultaneously burning and melting in my body. The radioactive material was coursing through my veins, and I felt a warm sensation all over my body from the outside in.

They discovered that I had DVT—deep vein thrombosis, which is just a fancy word for a blood clot in my vein, probably caused by the C-section. I was put on antibiotics and a daily injection of Clexane, a blood thinner, for the next few months.

I had always hated my hips growing up. I thought that they were disproportionately large for the rest of my body. Never had I been so thankful for the fattier parts of my body. The injections hurt like a bitch. But on the fattier parts they stung less. And so I spent the next few months rotating Clexane injections on my hips, where the extra fat absorbed the pain and suddenly became my friend after years of being my enemy.

The day before I was released as a patient for the second time in this hospital, I received a visit from one of the Russian doctors who had been responsible for removing my staples after my C-section. She remembered me. When she saw me in the women's hospital ward, she raised her hands to her cheeks. "Oh, no! Why are you here? What happened?" I told her about the DVT. "Oh, no! Practically everything that could have gone wrong went wrong!"

Well, I thought to myself, what can you do? Life is cruel. And I am so deep into this black hole of darkness and depression that I can't remember a time that I wasn't in this hospital, and I can't seem to picture any sort of future beyond this place.

CHAPTER 13

Drowning

My soul is anorexic,
Starving under the weight of reality.

Today's performance:
My body walks;
My soul crawls along beneath it like a shadow.
The whole world is a stage, isn't it?

I hate my life.
I lift my eyes to the heavens.
I bow; I pray on bended knee,
Begging for help.
But who can hear me?
I pound my fist into the ground, choke on my tears,
But no one is listening.

Is God this cruel?
My prayers float up into the nothingness,
And all I hear in return is silence.

Death can't be as cruel as this life.

CHAPTER 14

Privacy

My mood swings with your blood sugar level.
It's emotionally exhausting
To be so high and so low.

I don't know whether I stopped believing in God or whether I was so profoundly angry and so profoundly grateful that I could not process both feelings simultaneously: Do I pray to a god I don't believe in? A god I cannot trust? Is he nonexistent, or negligent and apathetic? Having such strong emotions on both sides of the bell curve was impossible to maintain for so long. I needed to let one side go. But which? And how?

I was alone with you for the first time today. Totally alone. You were almost four months old. They let me bring you with all of your machines down to the fifth floor to room five. So quiet and so beautiful. It only took fourteen weeks for me to get to be totally alone with my son. It was so perfect that I said a prayer, thanking God for letting me reach this momentous occasion.

I was finally able to hold you in the privacy of our own room. The weight of your body surprised me, and suddenly motherhood became even more real. Holding you in that moment, time stopped, suspended, just for us.

Then the glucose monitor beeped. Glucose low and dropping. The perfect moment was so transient. Shattered. Shoved back into the reality of medicine and beeping and monitors. So perfect, yet so gone.

CHAPTER 15

Sanity

THE CHAOS OF THE NICU is maddening. It's the beeping that really drives you mad. All the rows of babies, with all their monitors. *Beep, beep, beep.* Day after day in a dystopia, a storm of noise. As maddening as they are at first, the noises begin to fade into the background as the weeks go by. The day you come in and hear perfect silence is when you know you've lost it completely.

CHAPTER 16

Elana

Our next-door neighbors in the NICU had a daughter named Elana who is just about your age. The general rule for parents in the NICU was not to speak to another parent unless spoken to and not to look at anyone else's child. Everyone was encumbered with their own sad stories. When you were completely overwhelmed and beyond your capacity, sharing, commiserating, and asking questions about other patients didn't do anything but deplete you further.

We occupied the end of one of the rows in the intensive section of the NICU. Before you were released, you had to pass through one section for more highly intensive patients and two for less-intensive patients. Since we were on the inside of the row, we had a window on one side. It was sealed closed, so there was no fresh air, but at least we had a view. The other side was an aisle we shared with a young religious Jewish couple that couldn't have been older than twenty-three. I tried not to look over at their child, but it was hard. Babies generally don't look like anything when they are born, but if they are sick, the pain of seeing a newborn hooked up to tubes and needles is heartbreaking. It's easier to see your own child as a baby, not a patient, because he is yours.

I tried to mind my own business, but sometimes the mother's tears, sobs, and wailing broke through the wall I had built in my mind and the blinders I had put on my eyes. "Elana," she would moan, as if she were trying to wake her daughter from her coma. I can still hear her voice in my head.

I don't know what Elana's diagnosis was. I only knew it was dire. And then one morning, they wouldn't allow me into the NICU. Your row was blocked, and her bed was surrounded by white dividers. At first I didn't understand what was going on. Why couldn't I visit you? Were you all right? One of the nurses assured me that you were fine and told me to return in two hours.

Then it hit me. The thought sickens me even now as I write this.

Life is fragile, short, and cruel. Often to those who least deserve it.

May her memory be a blessing.

When I came back two hours later, it was as if nothing had ever happened, except for an empty, vacant bed next to yours. It would be filled by the end of the day with a new patient. The doctors told me not to worry and assured me that her case was very different from yours. Nonetheless, I held you tighter that night and prayed, like every other night, that I would get to keep you for another day.

CHAPTER 17

Waiting and Dreaming

I WILL WAIT.
I will wait.
I will wait
To live—
But when I do live,
When I am not walking around like a corpse whose soul is being tortured,
Who isn't living someone else's bad dream…

When I can live,
When we are free,
I promise myself that I will live my best life.
We will live life to its fullest.
But now I will wait,
I will hope,
And I will dream about our best life.

Things I miss most:
Quiet
Privacy
Fresh air
Sunshine
Fresh air
Quiet

CHAPTER 18

Dangerously Low

THE HOSPITAL WAS A FOGGY haze, and I felt like I was sleepwalking through my worst nightmare. What kept me most grounded was the strict schedule my breasts had me on. I was pumping every three hours, and when I didn't adhere to the schedule, the ache of milk reminded me that it was time to pump. A few times, I thought that I would quit pumping, but Safta, who is a pulmonologist by training, said that pumping was the only thing I could do medically for you. As far as modern medicine has come, doctors have not been able to replicate the nutrition and immunities passed on from mother's milk; formula doesn't even come close. So, every three hours, around the clock, I zipped on my pumping bra, hooked up the pump, and magically transformed into a milking machine. A woman's body is really a wondrous instrument, pleasing in its form but surprisingly utilitarian in its design.

One morning, I left the NICU briefly, took the elevator down to room five, and pumped. You were asleep, and your sugars were high. I told the nurse, a very thorough, trustworthy Russian nurse, that I would be back in a half hour. When I came back, you were covered in beads of white sweat, sucking on your tongue as if you had a pacifier. Lying on your side. Eyes wide open but in total silence.

As I sterilized my hands and slipped on my sterile gown, I noticed that something was wrong. I called the nurse. "What happened? What is wrong?" She turned around with concern and ran over to your bed. She wiped your sweat with a cloth and checked your sugar. The Accu-Check blood-glucose checker read 29. Dangerously low. A normal blood-sugar level is between 70 and 120. Anything below 60 is problematic. Twenty-nine is dangerous—like if you remain at that level for too long, your body will shut down, and you will go into a seizure. Many hyperinsulinemia babies have seizures. The hospital team had managed to prevent that thus far.

The nurse ran to administer a shot of glucagon—the "EpiPen" of sugars—to immediately increase your blood-sugar level. The nurse was visibly upset at herself; she said that she had just checked you and didn't know how you managed to drop so quickly. This was the disease, the condition—evil in its nature, serious in its effects, and instantaneous in its impact.

At least, Safta said, trying to comfort me, you weren't asymptomatic. And if you were ever to get that low again, I would be able to recognize your symptoms. From then on, whenever you started to drop, I would tap on your nose and say *low, low* so as to teach you how to communicate when your sugars were dropping.

Unfortunately and fortunately, this was your first gesture.

CHAPTER 19

Yearning for Answers

THE LAST FEW WEEKS HAD felt like we were flying blind, groping our way through the darkness on the medical front. We had a diagnosis but no cure. As I had learned, there are two different types of hyperinsulinemia, transient and permanent. Transient goes away quickly and unexpectedly, as if by magic. Permanent you can grow out of as an infant, or it can last until adolescence. Quite a long range of possibility there, but the good news was that it is a childhood disease; the pancreas rids itself of problematic cells and begins to regulate itself properly sometime before adolescence.

Of the permanent variety, there are two diagnosed types, focal and diffuse. Focal is where the problematic cells, the ones producing too much insulin and thus forcing the blood-sugar level down, are localized in one section of the pancreas. In diffuse, the problematic cells are located all across the pancreas. The difference here is that focal is operable, and diffuse is much harder to operate on. With focal cases, there is a general recommendation among the American medical community to operate and remove the localized section of problematic cells. Diffuse is still operable, but often surgery ends up removing up to 98 percent of the pancreas and ensuring diabetes for the rest of the patient's life.

A lot of *blah, blah, blah* with categories that don't really explain much. Solutions that don't solve much. Very little was clear cut. Many shades of gray. We had some big decisions to make, and if we didn't make them, they would be made for us.

Once your genetics came back, you were diagnosed with permanent hyperinsulinemia. We waited weeks to determine whether you had the focal or diffuse form. The scan that would determine that was not available at your current hospital, and so we were scheduled for the scan at a nearby hospital, the only one in Israel that performed the scan. Weeks of anticipation led up to the day of the scheduled scan, called an F-Dopa scan.

I had been wallowing in a pool of my own despair, searching for meaning, yearning for answers. This scan gave me hope. I hadn't felt hope since you were diagnosed. Hope for answers. Hope for direction. Our decisions at this specific junction would matter. If you had focal, we could go ahead with a planned surgery. If diffuse, we would have to determine what to do next, whether to go ahead with a surgery, a full pancreatectomy, or to try and manage your condition medically at home. This scan, this information, would help us make some decisions. Plan your future. Our future as a family.

The day of the scan we woke up early. An ambulance was scheduled to transfer us to the other hospital with a resident accompanying us, and then you would be returned "home," to your little giraffe in the NICU, in a matter of hours. You had been put on a glucose drip, as foods were forbidden twenty-four hours prior to the scan, and they left another IV in your little arm for the injection fluid for the scan. The injection fluid was dangerous and radioactive but the only way to perform the scan.

I was a ball of nerves that day. It was our absolute first time leaving hospital grounds with you, albeit to go to another hospital—but when you are in a constant state of crisis, all unknowns are terribly stressful. A marathon in a state of emergency dulls you to outside forces, but the stress manages to linger, seep into your subconscious, and traumatize your soul. So, at three and a half months, you rode in your first ambulance. Unfortunately, it wouldn't be your last. As we pulled into the new hospital, I noticed how familiar it looked. Same unfortunate, boring, depressing colors—white with a trim of some boring neutral color that made me want to puke. I know that to be a doctor or nurse, you must be very passionate about your calling, but something about the institution of a hospital manages to suck the lifeblood out of anyone inside it. No furniture, empty halls. God forbid someone should have a place to sit or sleep comfortably in the waiting room while watching over her loved ones.

We rolled you to the radiology department, where they performed the scans. As they led us down the hall, I noticed another couple with a four-year-old boy sitting on the plastic chairs in the waiting room. I saw them checking his blood-sugar level from his big toe, and I wondered if they were here to perform the same scan. They were.

What surprised me about this boy was how normal he looked. He wasn't hooked up to anything. No machines, no beepers, no ventilation. Just a normal little boy, running around the waiting room, full of energy, loath to sit on a chair. Jumping around, with a wild imagination, miming a fake sword to slay a dragon, rescuing a princess from her castle.

I wondered: Would you be that boy in a few years? Was there hope to be had? The mother and father of the four-year-old introduced themselves to us. They, too, had been in the NICU for what felt like a lifetime. They, too, had raised a boy with hyperinsulinemia through intensive treatment, monitoring, and care. I remember one thing specifically that the father said: that they had "the privilege of seeing their son get better." Would we too have that privilege?

When your life is so totally overwhelming that you can only take it day by day, hour by hour, even minute by minute sometimes, it is hard to try to envision the future. It is even harder to try to envision a positive future. But for a brief moment, his words cut through the fog in my heart, and I allowed myself to hope again, to dream, and to imagine a better future.

I paced the halls as they took you in for your scan. Not only did you have radioactive materials literally coursing through your veins, but they also needed to briefly put you under anesthesia so the scan could be performed. I was absolutely terrified, but they allowed us to watch through the window as the huge GE machine slid you through a circular tube, scanning, imaging. There were four or five screens behind the glass. All of a sudden, neon red, blue, green, and black danced across the screen. I wasn't an expert, but even if I had been, I don't think I could have made anything out of the scan being pieced together from the pixels of the screen. As the picture began to form, hope began to bubble again. Were these the answers we were looking for? We asked the specialist performing the scan her opinion of the results as they lit up the screen. She said that she couldn't tell offhand, and the scan had to be sent to specialists for conclusive results. It would take three weeks.

My heart sank. Another three weeks? We waited weeks to schedule the scan, and now more waiting. I could spend my whole life waiting. Waiting for answers. Waiting for a better tomorrow. At least now, I had a sliver of hope to hold onto as we waited another eternity.

Three weeks came and went with the beeping of the monitors in the NICU. Nothing seemed to change. Hyperinsulinemia—our diagnosis. Waiting—our treatment. Hoping—our solace. Until one day, a phone call came from the other hospital. Our results were in. The official transcript and images would be sent via mail to our current hospital.

The results: inconclusive.

As the attending spoke the words "inconclusive," a lump formed in my throat. My chest tightened. My eyes tried to fight back the tears. Why had I let myself hope? Why had I held on to the promise of more information, more knowledge, more anything to help us make an educated decision? I felt a huge wave of disappointment. We would have to make all of our decisions, all of our plans for a better future, with the current information we had. And that felt like very little. Big, life-changing decisions made on little slivers of information.

All the hope I had allowed myself dissipated in that moment. And I was left with nothing. Nothing. Nothing but fear and emptiness.

CHAPTER 20

Decisions and Data

Just another typical day in the NICU, but today the rotation changed. The head doctors switched, and Pompous was now in charge of the whole NICU.

We were doing OK up until today. We managed to get into a fairly regular schedule. They even let us take you out of the NICU for walks. For that, we were the envy of all the parents in the NICU. So between our daily schedule of injections every four hours, pumping every three hours, inhalations at 10:00 a.m. and 2:00 p.m., and physical therapy in the early afternoons, I managed to take you outside for a few breaths of fresh air and sunshine. All other medical tests—the echocardiograms, ultrasounds, and other major checks—were completely random and at the discretion of the specialists. Major surgeries were scheduled a few days in advance.

You had three major surgeries scheduled while we were there, and a fourth international surgery was scheduled for us in Germany, with another scan prior to surgery. First, they wanted to put in a central line so that it would be easier to take blood and do transfusions, but when they took you down to surgery, you turned white, your vitals became unstable, and they canceled the surgery and rolled you right back up. When your heart defect didn't close on its own, they scheduled a specialist from

Tel Aviv to come close it. This time they cleared out the room and sterilized your spot in the NICU. They said that this heart surgery could be performed at your bedside rather than in the operating room. So Abba and I waited outside, Abba with his prayer book, reading Psalms. I tried to pray, I did. But I needed a better distraction, so I helped the cleaning lady fold and sterilize equipment. It kept my hands busy and my mind occupied. Nothing better to clean the mind than menial labor. The third was a gastrostomy, where they replaced the feeding tube through your nose with a PEG tube. And your final surgery, a pancreatectomy, was scheduled with a specialist in Germany in three weeks. Ironic, isn't it? How your ancestors went to Germany to die, and we were going there to save your life.

As we prepared for your last surgery, we consulted with international specialists and debated the advantages and disadvantages. There is a split in the medical community on how to treat hyperinsulinemia. Israelis tend to recommend intensive, aggressive medical management until the childhood disease passes. Americans recommend surgery, specifically pancreatectomies—that is, removing part or most of the pancreas as early as possible. Pancreatectomies generally cure hyperinsulinemia, but new studies show that they almost guarantee diabetes later once the child reaches puberty. So, putting aside the actual financial considerations, there is a cost-benefit ratio to both methods. And since your initial scan was inconclusive, we didn't have any additional information to inform our decision.

We set a date for your surgery but hoped that it wouldn't have to come to that. However, as the days passed and the surgery and logistics needed to be set, we came down to the final count, needing to make a decision.

Having been in the NICU for four months, I quickly realized that all collective medical knowledge about each patient is lost and rebuilt with the rotation of the head doctors. Rather than reading each patient's medical history, babies are treated with a set of fresh eyes. The slate is wiped clean, and treatment begins anew. This is both a great opportunity to refresh and think creatively about each patient and at the same time a terrible opportunity to lose valuable knowledge and data.

NICUs are generally very good at treating early and sick babies aggressively and nursing them back to health in a matter of days or weeks, but we had been in this NICU for months now, and you were one of very few babies who seemed to be a permanent fixture. After expressing my frustration at the loss of your entire medical history during the first rotation change, I mobilized and built an Excel spreadsheet of your medical data and history. The staff might lose details of your history, but I would retain it, build upon it, be able to quickly recognize trends and correlations, and easily communicate it to your caretakers with charts and graphs.

In Israel, unlike in the U.S., patients are allowed access to their medical records. So, every night, Safta would pour over your medical records, translating them and consulting with her colleagues in the medical community. Other mothers would sit by their babies singing and praying. I would sit by your bed, inputting data into your Excel. I was sick of prayer, of hope. Those were too intangible, immaterial. I wanted numbers, graphs, logical explanations, answers. If God and your doctors couldn't give me any answers, maybe the data could.

CHAPTER 21

Pompous

TODAY WAS THE LOWEST OF the low. Pompous was in charge now, and even though we had four months of medical history in the NICU, he decided to start over.

In addition to your current medications, you had been on a concoction of mother's milk plus Nutramigen, a special lactose-sensitive formula, for the past few weeks. We had gone through the entire gamut of formulas, and after determining that you were lactose intolerant from the sheer volume of vomit you produced, we went through Similac, Materna, and Neocate before settling on Nutramigen. After charting your sugars on each formula, it was clear to me that Nutramigen was our best-bet solution. But no, Pompous decided to start over.

He demanded that you be put on a concentrated, milk-based Similac formula. It's a trick that NICU doctors use to pack on calories to preemies, and he thought that it would help keep your sugars up. He gave the order to your resident and nurse, and I saw your nurse start to argue with him. Israelis aren't big believers in hierarchy, so I saw her break rank and begin trying to share your long, long medical history and reaction to formula in the NICU. This particular nurse had been taking care of you for four months now, and I trusted her to know what was best for you. But Pompous disagreed. She came to me in secret to share his new plan to put you on Similac, and I was immediately frustrated at his incompetence, oversight, and lack of respect for the time we had spent tweaking your food to get it to the optimal mix—even though optimal, in this case, was far, far from perfect.

I pumped every three hours, avoiding dairy, and we spent months with the nutritionist evaluating formula options to minimize your vomiting and to maximize your sugars. He ignored all of this without a second thought, with just a look of disdain.

When I told the resident that we refused to go backward, that I refused to subject my son to a futile exercise that was destined to fail, she told Pompous to speak with me. I calmly told him that after months spent investing in your health and well-being, tweaking your food and medications, we could not afford to ignore history.

We launched into a tête-à-tête.

Me: "It is clear from past experience that my son has an intolerance to lactose. We tried all the formulas, and the dairy-based formulas increased his vomiting significantly, which obviously adversely affects his sugars."

Pompous pulled rank, looking down his nose at me: "You are a new mother, and I am a physician with twenty years of experience with babies. I recommend we take this course of action, and this is how we shall proceed."

Me, starting to get frustrated: "I understand that you have experience, but I have sat here to oversee my son's treatment for twelve hours a day the past four months. I live by his bedside. I know his treatment, symptoms, and side effects. I know my son and his medical history better than anyone. We have specialists from all over the world consulting on his condition. It would be imprudent to ignore his medical history and intolerance to milk. He has been through enough, and I cannot let you conduct this futile experiment on him."

Pompous: "You are emotional and cannot see the situation clearly. In my experience, it has helped many of my patients, and we will proceed with trying it on your son."

Me: "You are right. I am emotional, because this is my son. But this is a rare case. I will not allow you to throw out four months of medical history just because you started paying attention now. I have charted his sugars on each of these formulas." (I pulled up the chart on my iPhone.) "As you can see, his sugars were lowest on Similac compared to all of the other formulas, and highest on Nutramigen. I am emotional, but this is data. This is fact."

Pompous: "You do not have his best interests at heart because you are too emotional. You are interfering with your son's treatment, and he will suffer for it. If you continue to interfere with his proper treatment, I will no longer be able to treat your son."

My heart broke, and I tried to fight back the tears. Not have your best interests at heart? Interfering with treatment? Refuse to treat you? My mind raced.

I knew that I was right, but if I continued to engage in this conversation, I knew we would pay for it later. I ran out of the NICU, tears streaming down my face. I had worked so hard, tried so hard, to be a good mother, good nurse, good parent, good advocate, and here I was after four months of tireless work and complete dedication to your health, and here he was, Pompous, telling me that I was interfering and detrimental to your treatment.

I felt defeated. I found a hiding spot next to the service elevators. Slumped behind the garbage bin, I let my head fall into my open palms, and I began to sob.

After all of my hard work, trying to be strong, trying to do what was best for my family, I had been treated like garbage, and next to the discarded medications and dirty laundry, I had found my rightful spot in the hospital hierarchy.

CHAPTER 22

Pompous Postmortem

The next morning, Pompous came over to your giraffe. The conversation was strained. But I had a good night's sleep behind me, and I saw things a bit more clearly. From my previous experience working with megalomaniac dictators, I knew that there was only one way to deal with them. Power, logic, statistics, graphs, experience, attention to detail—none of these things speak to them. To get through, you need to appeal to their egos. As much as I believed I was right, I knew for a fact that for the next month, he was the dictator of the NICU, and he could make our lives hell. However, I also knew that as your parents and guardians, we had a legal right to the final say in your treatment, and since this was Israel, with a socialized medical system, he could not legally refuse to treat you without legal consequences and even jail time.

Our conversation went a little something like this:

Pompous: "Mrs. Hacohen, where is your husband?"

Me: "He is at work."

Pompous: "When will he be home?"

Me: "I dunno. Late."

Pompous: "Well, since he's not here, I will speak with you directly. We cannot properly treat your son when you are interfering with his treatment. I wanted to put him on Similac because it is high in sugar. I am a doctor, and this is not a simple case. You need to let me do my job, and going forward, I would request that you not interfere with his treatment. I know you are emotional because he is your son, but you don't know what is best for him. Good-bye."

Me: "You motherfucking motherfucker. I will kill you. I will slit your tires. I will rape, burn, and pillage until you have nothing left."

OK. I didn't really say that last bit. But I wanted to. I stared directly into his eyes as if my retinas were burning a hole into his chest and melting him into oblivion. I bit my tongue and cursed him to the seventh circle of hell in my mind.

I thought it was best that way. I was a mother now, and however I felt personally, I was playing a long game, and I wasn't playing it alone. I was playing it for my family. It might not have been the right thing to do, but it was surely the smart thing.

Since our conversation went so swimmingly in the morning, I thought that discussion would be our last. Imagine my surprise when he called me into his office that afternoon.

What could we possibly have left to talk about? I waited outside and then knocked on his door. As I entered, I reminded myself that patience was a virtue and that being smart was more important than being right.

Oh, boy. Here we go again, I thought as I took a seat across from his desk.

Pompous: "Please take a seat. Well, tell me how you see his condition and care up until now."

Hmm, I thought to myself, a promising beginning. He is including me in the dialogue and discussion about treatment. I thought it best to try to give as medical a perspective as I could. To him, we weren't talking about my son. My firstborn, one and only child. To him, you were a patient.

Me: "Well, my son was born in week thirty-eight. He was diagnosed at birth with hyperinsulinemia and presented with pulmonary hypertension, fat necrosis, and a host of other issues. He was treated with Glucagon, Sandostatin, and Diazoxide for his low blood sugar in addition to continuous food via feeding tube.

He overcame the pulmonary hypertension and started breathing on his own about a month ago. The fat necrosis he also overcame in week four; no one is sure why. Then he presented with impaired liver function and a large defect in his heart, which was closed via surgery. A gastrostomy was performed to assist with his continuous feeds.

We were lucky that he was diagnosed so quickly, but your consulting endocrinologist is following not leading. She took him off Diazoxide only after we brought in a secondary medical opinion report from the Children's Hospital of Philadelphia (CHOP). The CHOP report recommended discontinuing Diazoxide as the medical literature indicated it was ineffective medication for him based on the genetics. She submitted the paperwork to request a continuous glucose monitor only once we, the family, advocated for it at the behest of other medical professionals. She has visited him, her only NICU patient, once or twice a week at most during our entire four month stay, even during periods when he was quite unstable.

In spite of her mediocrity, he went from being on twenty medications a day and now is only on glucagon injections six times a day and continuous food. We are very familiar with his regimen now. Our lives in the hospital have, for better or worse, become habitual, and we don't see any additional potential for a change in treatment beyond the international surgery we were preparing for.

You guys have done a great job getting him better. We know that he is a very complicated case and a tricky patient. Having said that, my husband and I feel that treatment-wise, we've hit a brick wall. We are ready to go home and for you to release us and for us to care for him at home prior to his international surgery. These additional last-ditch efforts are just that. Small tricks to try to stabilize his sugars. We have agreed and done most of them already in the first few months we were here. We have been here four months, and every time the head of the NICU changes, we circle back, and it's as if you are starting treatment all over again.

"We have four months of data that we have collected. That is being ignored. See this chart. This chart is an Excel of his sugars going back four months, each on a different formula. As you can see, his sugars were lowest on the Similac and Neocate and highest on the Nutramigen. In addition, after careful observation, my husband and I believe that he has an allergy to milk. He has strong reflux as part of his condition, but he throws up much more often on the milk-based formulas. We can't repeat all the small tricks we've already tried to stabilize his sugars."

Pompous (condescendingly): "Well, it's very nice that you took the time to make those graphs But you don't have any experience as a doctor. I have over twenty years of experience as a pediatric physician."

But I know my son better than you do, you fucking asshole. And, by the way, we are arguing about food here, not medication. You don't have to be a neuroscientist to figure out food. This is purely trial and error, and it was already tried!

Pompous: "And, madam, what you call tricks, we call therapeutic care."

Arrrr, I will slice you. I will slice your tires and then your wrists.

Me: "Look, as I said, you guys have done a great job. My intention is not to get in your way. We have the same objective—to get my son better. We are on the same team."

Pompous: "If you continue to interfere with his treatment, I will have to recuse myself from his case."

Me: "If you wish. That is your prerogative. We would prefer to have a senior doctor on his case, but if you don't feel comfortable, I understand. I think that we can work together. We are on the same team."

Pompous: "Well, I have decided that we will not try a new formula. We can continue to work together unless you get in the way again."

Bite your tongue, Raissa. You got what you wanted. Leave before you say anything else.

You should choke and die, and I will spit on your grave. The words were forcing themselves out of my throat like vomit. And like a good girl, I swallowed them up with a plastic smile seeped in distain.

Me: "Thank you for your time."

CHAPTER 23

Hail Mary

After that episode, your abba and I knew that this was the best that this hospital could do. We were grateful for the great deal that they had done to get you healthy up until now, but as we looked forward and longed for home, we knew deep down that these were not the doctors that would get us there.

The hospital endocrinologist had resigned herself, for lack of any better options, to sending us to Germany for a pancreatectomy to remove most of your pancreas. She was so resigned that she was only visiting you once or twice a week, as if we had already transferred care to your international surgery team. Never mind that fact that with continuous food and multiple shots, we didn't think that you were stable enough to withstand another surgery, let alone an international flight to Europe.

This was our last chance. A last Hail Mary before the surgery. As parents, we couldn't live with ourselves unless we had exhausted all other options prior to flying.

We gave Safta the mission of finding a new doctor, a new hospital, a partner with whom we could discuss our dilemmas and challenges and plan your future. I only wish we had found him sooner.

Dr. Smith was everything we had been looking for but hadn't yet found in a physician. He wasn't a god, but he was the closest thing to it that I have ever encountered. He was an experienced endocrinologist, well respected and connected in the international community. He had both the patience and courage to make bold medical decisions and see them through, but he lacked the ego and arrogance of his peers. He was flexible and adaptable enough to change course if a treatment wasn't working, and most important, he was a true partner in navigating the course of your treatment. He acknowledged that we were your primary caregivers and consulted with us on his every move, pushing us when necessary, listening when important. Straddling the delicate line of leadership artfully. The best doctors know that medicine is more of an art than a science.

CHAPTER 24

The Hospital Switch

We neglected to tell the hospital NICU team of our transfer until the day of. Maybe not the most generous gesture but probably the most strategic, since we wanted to secure the utmost care for you until our departure. We notified them that morning. Most of the staff members were shocked; some were even offended. But I think the staff that we worked most closely with understood. The current resident on your case even said that we had to feel secure that we were exhausting all options prior to your international surgery, and that as a parent she would have done the same thing.

I packed up room five in garbage bags and said good-bye and good riddance to our home of the past four months. No love lost there. The NICU staff recommended that we—or rather, they compelled us to—transfer you to the hospital via ambulance. So at four months old, you traveled in your second ambulance, and at twenty-nine years old, I traveled in mine. It was only your second time off hospital grounds, but you never would have known it. The lull of the engine put you fast asleep.

As a gesture of goodwill, one of the senior doctors offered to accompany us for the ambulance ride, and for that I was grateful. They carefully moved you from your giraffe onto a gurney and into the ambulance, still hooked up to travel monitors and continuous food and medication. I remember the ride like it was yesterday. How everything in the ambulance was packed in and secured so it wouldn't fall off the walls, how the gurney snapped into place, the seat belts on the side. Were all ambulance drivers terrible drivers? I figured that this one was because he was used to rushing from place to place. We weren't particularly in a rush, but he drove swiftly with the lights on, siren blaring, parting traffic like the Red Sea.

When we arrived at our destination, I thanked our accompanying doctor for all her time and attention. She gave me a big smile and a bear hug.

CHAPTER 25

A New Beginning

After so little sleep; exhaustion begins to weigh you down. Running a mental marathon is hard, especially because you don't know where the finish line is. You can't tell where the milestones are, so it's impossible to gauge whether you're ahead or behind, close to the finish line or only in the first mile. Exhausting because you don't know when to push harder or reserve your strength. You can only run the ten feet in front of you and hope that you're doing well enough. But there are no grades, no bonuses, no telltale signs that you are doing OK.

This was a hard decision—moving, I mean, because it wasn't necessarily the right move. I thought it was the smart move, but I thought we'd only be able to tell in hindsight if it was the right one.

One of the senior doctors said something really sweet before we transferred hospitals. Maybe I misunderstood her, because she did have a very thick Russian accent in Hebrew. But she said that you have been through a lot and that you weren't lucky by a lot of parameters, since you've had to overcome so much. But you did luck out when it came to your parents. I thought that was really sweet and touching.

We were now in the intermediate pediatric unit at hospital number two. Dr. Smith came by to talk to us, and he called the nurses twice after his visit to check up on you and hear about your blood-sugar levels. Also, the head of the unit asked for your full medical report to read and gave me her cell number and e-mail. I thought that you would get better attention here. It was weird because it was so quiet—it didn't feel normal. No beeping and bleeping, and every time your saturation went down—it was fine; the machine just wasn't reading it correctly—the nurse came over straightaway. One second later, like magic.

I did miss all the characters of the NICU and their ridiculous ways; they had become our family once we'd become parents. But I thought that this would be a fresh start. This was a much better fit for you. For us. And for the first time ever, I got to fall asleep next to my son. Quiet. Relatively quiet. Alone. Relatively alone. A semblance of privacy in a room with three walls and a curtain. I said a prayer to thank God for getting us to this moment in time.

Part II

CHAPTER 1

Misery Loves Company

In the midst of it all, I received an e-mail from a close friend who had herself become a patient temporarily to undergo a major surgery. I wrote to her:

To my dearest friend,

I am not sure where to begin. When did life get so complicated? I remember a time, not so long ago, when our biggest problems were what classes to take and whom to date. I feel like I've aged to about one hundred over these past few years. Even though the days of our youth aren't so far away, they feel like an eternity.

Firstly, I want you to know that I love you, and I know that you have the strength, courage, and grace to face this head-on. I have all the confidence in you in the world. I know that it's hard to stay positive in the face of such uncertainty, but if anyone can, it's you!

We have had a rough time over here as well. We have a scheduled date to fly to Germany for my son's surgery on January 20. There is a week of testing, and surgery is the following week if all tests go as planned. In the meantime, we just switched hospitals. It was a tough decision, but ultimately my husband and I felt that we knew the doctors' treatment plan was to maintain him until the surgery, and we thought that we owed it to our son and ourselves to get a fresh pair of eyes before we went to surgery. He is improving, but it still looks like surgery is our only option right now. It's hard to believe that we've been living in hospitals for the past four months, but I really think it's the best thing right now, so I'm just trying to get through each day.

That said, I do have a few coping strategies that I thought I might share in the hope that they help you, too.

1) Listen to the music but not the words. The therapist I started seeing mentioned this one to me. I was feeling like everyone had to put in their two cents about how we were handling the situation and to see how we were doing, and it was just awful. One nameless woman asked me after my emergency C-section, "How are your bowel movements?" Hello? I know that she meant well, and what she really meant to say was, how are you doing and are you taking care of yourself during this whole ordeal? But it came out as verbal diarrhea. So when you can, try to listen to the music but not the words of your friends and loved ones. No one else can ever really know what you are going through.

2) I think that the uncertainty is the hardest part. Try to create habit and familiarity whenever you can. Here are some of my coping strategies for hospitalization:

A) Atmosphere: Try to bring with you things that are familiar and relaxing.

- Comfort Food: I brought my favorite kind of really expensive tea that I never usually treat myself to and barrels of Trader Joe's peanut butter (because it reminds me of home and is a true comfort food).
- Music: Nothing sets a mood better than music. I must have listened to the same three relaxation mixes on 8tracks thousands of times in the past few months. It helps take you back to another place with good memories.
- Sight: There were no good windows or fresh air in our hospital, so I look at photos of the outdoors on my phone—so depressing, I know :). Pack some gossip mags or other light reading. I am sure that reading will be tough, but looking at photos or even old albums might be fun.
- Smell: They don't really let you burn candles, but if you can bring something that smells like home or freshness, that is helpful.
- Planning: This helps the control freak in all of us. I have been planning to live my best life for the past four months, what I would do, where I would go. Maybe you can plan a workout regimen or training for a marathon, something to look forward to once you've recovered completely. Even though you have to take one day at a time, it helps to dream big.

B) Feel your feelings when you feel them.

- This seems obvious, but after my C-section, everyone was just trying to cheer me up, and I was really upset and disappointed and had so many other feelings going on. Someone came to visit me, and she told me that I just had to allow myself to experience all those feelings instead of fighting them, and then they would just wash away. And then they did.

- After you have worked through some of your feelings, start trying to treat yourself like a person and not a patient, and ask others to do the same. My mom spent so much time trying to help me and baby me, it actually made me feel more helpless and less independent. Be clear with others what your needs are.
- There are two types of people who can be helpful to you during this time. I call them gladiators and cheerleaders. If people fall outside of these categories, don't spend your valuable energy on them right now. A gladiator is just someone who can do your bidding without questions. A lot of people will have many opinions on what is best for you. Only you can know, and you should lean on the people who can respect that. Cheerleaders are people who can't actually help with tasks but just with emotional support. I found that pity is the absolute worst thing that someone can feel, and it makes you feel a thousand times worse, but when someone says you are doing great and just cheerleads along the sidelines, it really can make a difference.

C) Recovery

- When you are ready, push yourself to wear real clothes. Those hospital gowns that don't close in the back are the worst, and they make you feel like a patient and not a person.
- Try to organize it so that you eat as little hospital food as possible. Hospital mush makes you feel like a patient, and I found that just getting takeout from a nearby café or restaurant can make all the difference. We were lucky to have friends and family prepare fresh-cooked meals and deliver them to us every day for the past few months.
- When you are ready, accept visitors. I had a really hard time with this one. I found that the best visitors were

my work colleagues, because in my spare time I didn't want to talk about my situation but rather hear about something more distracting and less heavy. You may feel differently, but family and close friends were actually the most draining visits.

- If you can, try to get a little sunshine and a bit of fresh air every day. Probably not so feasible during the winter, but even just sitting by a window helps.
- This one is also from my therapist: any problem that can be solved with money is a good one. This becomes so crystal clear when you are dealing with an illness. If you are encountering any issues that can be solved with money, throw some money at the problem and make it go away. You have enough on your plate right now.

3) Sheryl Sandberg, COO of Facebook, said in her book, *Lean In*, that "the most important decision you will make in your whole career is who your partner is." I think this is true for life in general. I couldn't have gotten to this point without my husband. Whenever I felt I was stumbling in this unbearably long medical marathon, I felt like he put my arm over his shoulder and carried me along with him. I am glad that you have your husband and your family with you. Always keep your A team close by; no one else matters.

I love you, and if there is anything I can help with, please let me know. If you ever want to talk, let me know. I won't bug you, since I feel like you are probably overwhelmed by phone calls and e-mails, but know that if you just want to talk or want someone to listen, I am always here for you at any time, day or night.

As for us, there is still a lot of uncertainty. I feel like every time I prepare myself emotionally, the foundation collapses under my feet, and the tectonic plates are constantly moving. (It's an emotionally draining version of Dance Dance Revolution.) My son's condition has been getting more stable week by week. So much so that the tentative plan is that they are thinking of releasing us next week, and his doctors are even considering postponing the surgery. I don't want to get my hopes up too high yet.

My son's favorite songs are "The Ants Go Marching" and "Little Bunny Foo Foo." I find that the repetitiveness of the songs and marches just reminds you that you just have to keep putting one foot in front of the other every day, and just doing that makes you a very brave person.

I love you.

Your gladiator and cheerleader,
Raiss

CHAPTER 2

Preparing for Home

Last week I wrote a list of things I missed most. The list goes as follows:

Quiet
Privacy
Fresh air
Sunshine
Fresh air
Quiet

Preparing to come home was an incredible milestone. It was almost as awesome as it was terrifying. We would finally have our own time together, our own space as a family to just be. To just grow. To just enjoy each other's company without all of the other patients, nurses, doctors, and staff in the NICU participating, watching, observing us. It was what we had waited and worked for such a long, long time. Four and a half months is a long time to be away from home, in a sterile environment with crisp lab coats and rubber gloves, white walls and fluorescent lights that are permanently lit, no privacy, no quiet, no control.

So long, hospital, I said to myself—I will not miss you. Not one bit. I will forget you as quickly as I can in my mind and in my soul, and we will only now begin to build the type of childhood and the type of life that we wanted as a family.

Yet at the same time, I was terrified. We were but two parents. No medical training beyond the past four and a half months. You had a staff of fifteen trained professionals at your service at all hours. Why should we be able to care for you better than them? Because we are your parents and we love you, we would do our best, and that was all we could ask for.

CHAPTER 3

So Close

Home felt so close yet so far. Every additional day at the hospital sucked the breathless life out of us. A prison with wardens in white coats. You never really consider mobility a privilege until you lose it. And so we prepared to go home. A home that had been uninhabited for the past five months.

The first step was to stock everything. Machines: Kangaroo for feeding, monitor for heart rate and saturation at night. And meds—we practically built our own internal pharmacy. Our last week in the hospital, they sent us home for a few hours for a "dry run." I was so excited and so nervous at the same time. I packed everything we could possibly need. I remember reading the *Baby Whisperer* many months back while I was still pregnant, and she says that you should introduce your baby to its new home. Go room by room, explaining and touring your home. I had waited for so long to do this. So long to sleep in my own bed, in my own room, with your abba and you by my side.

I remember strapping you into your car seat for the first time. It felt almost forbidden, as if we were stealing you away, since we had never been allowed out before. We drove with the windows down and music blasting like we were sixteen-year-olds going on a long road-trip adventure. Even though it was a fifteen-minute ride home, it was to a world we had long forgotten. Our normal lives. Our home. Our bed. Our couch. Our sheets. Our food. Our home. With peace and quiet, privacy, no one observing our every move.

As we drove home with the windows down and music up, I noticed a beeping. Hmmm...What could it be? It turns out that the Kangaroo machine, which fed you continuous food and kept your sugars high, is a very sensitive machine. It was made for the monotony and immobility of hospitals. Every bump, every turn set it off, and it stopped, waiting for manual reactivation. So what was supposed to be our first magnificent adventure turned into a very stressful car ride that seemed to drag on forever, as I cradled your Kangaroo and manually reactivated it every time it began to beep.

And finally, we were home. I opened the door and wanted to give you the grand tour, but the lull of the car engine had put you to sleep. And you never wake a sleeping baby. So I let my OCD side run free, and I began unpacking and organizing your medical supplies and medications, making sure that we were properly stocked for our final discharge from the hospital.

I organized the house with one central location for all of your paraphernalia, and I put little pockets of meds and supplies in each room for urgent situations. As the weight and enormity of the responsibility of going home started to sink in, my OCD rose proportionately. Instead of relaxing at home for the first time in months, I began cleaning and scrubbing, organizing and reorganizing with the vigor of a woman possessed by Mr. Clean.

You woke up just as we had to head back to the hospital for the night. We got in the car and said, "Farewell but see you soon," to our home. As we drove back to the hospital, I heard another kind of beep, not the Kangaroo this time but your CGM, a continuous glucose monitor that we call your iPhone. It monitors your sugars, and yours were dropping quickly. As I turned off the beeping monitor, my heart leapt into my throat. Oh my God. Where was your glucagon, the EpiPen of sugars that I needed to administer urgently?

Nowhere in sight. I had been so busy unpacking and organizing all your medications at home that in my OCD haze, I had forgotten about the car ride. I knew that we had a supply at the hospital, but I hadn't taken into consideration the ride back. FUCK. FUCK. FUCK.

We sped back to the hospital, and I felt like the biggest failure in the world. The first three hours with full responsibility for you, and I had failed. Failed as a mother, as a nurse, as a pharmacist. How could I possibly be entrusted with your care at home?

We ran back to your hospital room, and I rushed to the medication corner, where they dispensed drugs and only nurses were allowed. I grabbed ten glucagon. I only needed one, but the nine extra were for in case I fucked up again. One went in my purse. One in your diaper bag. One in the car, et cetera. As I began calculating in which additional locations I could place your glucagon, the head nurse ran up to me and scolded me for going into the drug corner without a trained staff person.

My emotions overcame me, and I burst into tears. Tears for my failure, tears over the trepidation and fear for what was to come, and tears for whether I could be entrusted in the future with such a precious treasure outside the walls of this hospital.

CHAPTER 4

Home

Now in the sanctuary of our own home, the routine was as follows:

6:00 AM: Sildenafil
8:00 AM: Prepare Nutramigen formula with Polycose and corn flour in appropriate proportions
Noon: vitamin D, Sildenafil, Amlodipine
6:00 PM: Sildenafil
Midnight: Sildenafil, Amlodipine, Nexium, Euthorox

Switch needle for glucagon pump every six to eight hours.
Provide continuous food 24/7 via Kangaroo.
Administer glucagon shots as needed for hypoglycemia.
Keep pumping every four to six hours.

So busy being a doctor and a nurse and a milk machine.
No time to be a mother.

We were now mobile, but every trip outside was an ordeal. We'd have to pack enough milk for the journey. Unclip your Joey (the Kangaroo's more durable, compact cousin), the continuous food-delivery machine. Bring all the bags downstairs.

Put you in the stroller. Rehook your Joey. Cover you with the right blankets and throw-up cloths to strategically cover your machines. Tuck in your glucagon pump to your clothes. Tuck your blood-glucose monitor on your side. And then we were ready to go.

One time we bumped into String Bean in a French café next to our house. "Wow," she said. "He looks fantastic. He's so big, and he's no longer hooked up to anything! What a miracle!" We smiled and showed her how we had packed in and hooked up the Joey to the stroller, carefully threading the tube through the back to the front of the stroller and hooking you up strategically so that the machine and tubing weren't pulling and could function properly. She was shocked. And it was just an average day for us, taking a trip out to a café.

CHAPTER 5

Back to the Hospital

WE HEADED BACK INTO THE hospital after two months at home. You were getting your percutaneous endoscopic gastrostomy tube (PEG) replaced. The initial PEG takes two months to set, and then they replace it with a more stable piece. I hoped that this was another step in the right direction. The procedure, which also involves inserting a fiberoptic scope into the throat, would also give the doctors a chance to see what was wrong with your vocal cords. Had they been damaged by surgery? By the anesthesia? By all of your vomiting? Or was it something else that was preventing you from vocalizing anything louder than a whisper? If the procedure went smoothly, Dr. Smith wanted us to stay for another couple of days to try a new drug, Sandostatin, again.

When we were in the NICU, you were much more stable on the Sandostatin, but it was discontinued due to liver damage. But the liver damage had since healed itself, and the problem could have been attributed to a number of other medications you were on at the time. So, best case, the Sandostatin would now have no effects on your liver and keep your sugars much more stable. A majority of children with your condition are on Sandostatin, and if it worked, it could change our lives, as it was much easier to manage than glucagon.

The Sandostatin pump would need to be switched every three days, as opposed to every four to six hours on the glucagon. My life was a series of numbers with the glucagon. Sugar: eighty-three. Sugar: seventy-eight. Sugar: sixty-five. Maybe on the Sandostatin, I would have a few moments of reprieve away from your sensor, which dictated our lives right then. When we slept, when we awoke. When we ate, when I pumped. Your sugars needed to be constantly monitored and stable enough to complete each activity. Your abba and I were getting used to the exhaustion, but taking turns keeping your sugars up was a heavy load to bear. I felt the weight of responsibility on my shoulders every waking and sleeping moment.

It was hard to believe that we'd been parents for six months already. Six months of switching off duties hour by hour. And as slowly as those hours had passed, they'd also gone by really quickly. You were just full of smiles and laughs. Your baby laugh was not like anything in this world. It just melted away all the hurt and frustration and despair. You loved to dance and snuggle. We danced together to the Beatles, Adele, Florence and the Machine, and Simon and Garfunkel. You loved it. You were talking, too. It was all gobbledygook, but it was amazing nonetheless. I was so proud of you for hitting these huge developmental milestones and so thankful for all the good times. I hoped the worst was behind us.

The road back to the hospital as an inpatient was ridden with anxiety, emotional exhaustion, and psychological torment, but I would have done anything for you, my darling boy. Anything for you. Anything for our family. It was, at the very least, comforting to know that we would only be there for a limited time. And so I packed our bags and put on my brave face, because that was what my family needed. A brave mother.

But it was your bravery and the bravery of your abba that inspired me to be brave.

CHAPTER 6

PEG Switch

The PEG switch went smoothly. But wow, I did not miss the hospital at all. I had forgotten how exhausting it was to advocate for your child, their patient, every hour of every day. To make sure the doctors have the full picture and not just their little piece of the puzzle.

First of all, you kicked out your IV from your foot in the middle of the night. As I predicted. You needed to fast for your PEG switch, and since you were on continuous feedings, they put you on a D10 IV overnight, a drip IV of pure sugar. So at 6:00 a.m., they had to put a new one in, and then we waited until they admitted us to the gastroenterology unit at 11:00 a.m. The procedure had been scheduled for 8:00 a.m. Why did they even bother wearing watches? If you can't keep time, you should lose your watch privileges.

When we were admitted, the gastro doctors came to talk to us. "We are just going to swap it out," they said.

"No, the plan is that while you are in there, you need to do a laryngoscopy to see that everything is OK," we reminded them assertively.

From their point of view, they were minimizing risk by making the procedure quicker (and less thorough), since they were worried about your sugar dropping. They were planning to do their task as efficiently as possible, but we needed them to be effective, too. We saw the whole picture and had to advocate to ensure that they looked at you from a holistic diagnostic perspective. You always need to advocate for the bigger picture. Make sure the doctors know the key facts. Repeat them incessantly until they start correcting you, because they don't always have the full picture in the patient chart, and sometimes they barely have time to glance at it at all.

Anyway, your esophagus and stomach lining—everything looked fine. But they took biopsies of your esophagus to send to the lab, only because we advocated.

Then we got back to your hospital room, and the other two patients had been discharged. Hallelujah! A moment of privacy amid the chaos. As if a stupid dinky curtain afforded you any privacy. And since the other two patients had moved, we could move to the window seat! Double bonus, since these windows actually opened, so we had fresh air and sunshine. Hallelujah! It's the small pleasures that you really learn to appreciate.

But what now? No Sandostatin, you say?

"But we are staying hospitalized specifically for the Sandostatin trial," I stammered.

What, no one ordered it? Only tomorrow? Such bullshit. You literally have to shove your way through this bureaucratic system in order to get comprehensive healthcare. Well, fuck you and please order the Sandostatin for tomorrow morning. We want to go home.

CHAPTER 7

An Experiment of Hope

Freedom seems so close that you can taste it.
Maybe we can go on vacation.
Maybe I can go back to work.
Maybe we can sleep a full night.

Alas, the evil gods of Sandostatin,
Shining down on your sugars
While burning through your liver—

Experiment over. Back to glucagon.
Maybe this time the gods of glucagon will be better to us?

CHAPTER 8

Lucky

Even though the experiment was a failure, we felt lucky. Very, very lucky. I had the best husband in the universe and the strongest little warrior in the world.

Day three of our Sandostatin experiment, they called me over to see if I could help another baby with hyperinsulinemia. No one knew how to hook up the baby's pump. Not the father, not the staff. So I put in a new needle. Then half an hour later they called me to fix the reservoir. What? The rules were that you weren't even supposed to look at other people's babies, let alone touch them. It felt really weird to be the resident expert in hyperinsulinemia/insulin pumps in the hospital.

This baby did not look well cared for. He was huge and maybe had already had a seizure or two due to low blood sugar. So sad.

We were lucky that you were diagnosed early and treated properly. Not all hyperinsulinemic babies are so lucky.

We were lucky to have each other. And we were blessed to have you.

CHAPTER 9

Despair

WHAT A TERRIBLE FEW DAYS we had at home with your sugars. I was sitting all day at your side delivering glucagon boluses to boost your sugars. And I had no idea what was going on. What caused this change? And again my depression sank to despair.

I am so sorry that I cannot protect you.
I have failed as a parent over and over,
And it feels so terrible to feel powerless—
To be reactive, not proactive.

I feel like we regressed a few months in the past two days—
Hypos every two hours—
And I am struggling to keep up,
To send your sugars back up,
To return the ball to the other side of the court.
Your hypos are faster and more frequent.
I am struggling for a diagnosis or explanation so I can fix it.

God, tell me how.
Everything is in your hands.
I am powerless.
Please protect my son.
Please help me protect him.

CHAPTER 10

Data and Discovery

I WAS VERY PROUD OF myself today. After a few emotionally and physically exhausting days, I felt like we were back on track.

I was racking my brain to try to figure out what had changed to cause our difficult string of days, so I consulted with Dr. Safta, your primary doctor and grandma. I mentioned that this week we stopped the medication Amlodipine completely and asked if that could have an effect. Well, darling, Dr. Safta thought my differential diagnosis was very interesting.

Differential diagnosis is just fancy doctor-speak for the other options of what the problem could be aside from your first guess. It's one of those words that gets you in the club, getting doctors to talk to you on a peer level. Like when you use terms like *due diligence*—that is, homework—or *liquidity*, the ability to convert assets to cash, with financiers. It helps them realize that they are allowed to speak with you on their level. Dr. Safta taught me that.

Anyway, back to the Amlodipine. I spoke to your primary endocrinologist, Dr. Smith, and told him that was the only medical change we made this week. I asked whether it could it be a factor. He said that we should try putting you back on it and see what happens. Well, it turned out that Amlodipine, which they put you on for high blood pressure, is also a calcium channel blocker, controversial in the medical literature as to whether it can affect sugars. But let me tell you, you were an angel baby with your sugars ever since we went back to it. Superstable. I was really despairing yesterday, but today I was awarding myself an honorary doctorate. My title, henceforth, would be Dr. Chief Snuggle Officer.

I realized in the NICU that medicine is more of an art than a science. There is a lot more trial and error than they let on. The problem with doctors is that they tend not to treat each medication or treatment as a separate variable. Something isn't working, you feel worse, so in reaction, they change the whole treatment plan instead of isolating each variable to measure its effect. There should be a course in big data, variables, and methodology in medical school. We currently have so much data in health care, every patient is producing hundreds and thousands of data points every hour. They should learn how to use the data to diagnose and treat patients.

In the meantime, in the nearly seven weeks we had been back home, we got to use our calculated methodology of isolating and changing one variable at a time. It was very apparent that the Amlodipine was the only variable that had changed in the previous few days.

You were stable, and I could breathe a big sigh of relief. I now worshipped at the feet of the god of Amlodipine.

CHAPTER 11

A Chance Meeting with Vienna

It was weeks before your planned eye surgery. You were eight months old and wearing glasses all the time. We were rotating putting a patch over your eye as instructed by your eye doctor. Sometimes people who passed us on the street would peer into your stroller and say, "Glasses? So young?" I would just smile, nod, and continue on our way, laughing to myself that glasses were the least of what we were dealing with. As far as I was concerned, they were an accessory trumped by far more significant, urgent, and life-threatening health concerns. The glasses were merely ornamental, and truth be told, they became part of your personal style.

We were on an outing in the neighborhood, and we stopped on the sidewalk to admire the rose bushes when an older woman walked by. She must have been in her eighties or nineties. She stopped by your stroller to peek in. "Glasses?" she asked. I rolled my eyes and nodded politely in her direction. "So young?" she said.

"Uh-huh," I replied, wanting to keep on our way without being too rude.

She startled me by taking my hand. “When I was a young girl in Vienna,” she began, “I was four and I couldn’t see very well, my eyes were partially crossed. I was scheduled for an eye surgery, and then the Nazis came. They took away all our glasses and canceled my surgery.” She turned over her wrist to show me her number, tattooed on her forearm. She stopped her story there. Her eyes were teary, and I could tell that it was too hard for her to continue.

“He is very lucky to have glasses so young, and it is good that you are dealing with it so early. He will go to surgery, and everything will be fine. He will live a long life,” she said with certainty. She squeezed my hand and continued on her way.

I was taken aback by her story. It reminded me of a different time and place, where people like us wouldn’t have had access to health care and doctors like we did seventy years later. It reminded me that many people even today don’t have this kind of access to health care.

Her certainty comforted me, and suddenly this surgery, your eye surgery, became less daunting. For a moment, I was able to hold on to the hope that everything would be all right.

CHAPTER 12

Eye Surgery

And here we are again. Inpatient. Another waiting room. Another lifetime of waiting. Waiting to breathe deeply. Waiting to know that you are safe.

I am so sick of waiting, of feeling defeated. I have no more tears to cry; the well is dry. No more energy to feel. I am empty. Running on empty is difficult, but I assume that most moms do it often. Motherhood almost demands it.

I know now that I have no control, no influence over the outcome of events. That used to be an overwhelming feeling—that I have no control—but I have made my peace with it. I have struggled with it, and it has defeated me.

So I am waiting once again. Waiting.

CHAPTER 13

Grandpa Sid

Grandpa Sid was an amazing man. He was twelve went he and his family left Germany on the last boat, the *Aquitania*, allowed out in 1939. He grew up in New York and enlisted in the army during World War II to go back and fight the Nazis. He never spoke about that dark time in history. He never spoke about the war.

He was a loving and proud grandfather. He loved the arts and music. He made sure that his grandchildren were exposed to culture: dance, music, theater. He was eighty-seven when he passed away. He was still playing softball and volunteering at the local hospital up until his death.

He was the first grandparent I lost. You were eight months old.

I flew to New York for two days to attend his funeral. I remember the chazzan, the choirmaster, of his synagogue giving his eulogy. He spoke of Grandpa Sid's love of music, his joy for life, and his ability to appreciate the beauty in life. I regret that he never got to meet you in person. You Skyped with him a few times, but he never got to hold you, to hug you, to kiss you. I miss him, and I wish that you had the privilege of meeting him, too, of learning from him, of loving him as I did.

His memory will be a blessing, and I will always remember how proud he was of you, of us, even from very far away. I wish for you that you inherit his love of life, his love of music, his strength, and his ability to see beauty and humor in the most unlikely of places.

CHAPTER 14

PEG

In the middle of the night, at 2:00 a.m., your abba woke me. "Raissa, wake up," he said in a stern tone. He never spoke sharply, so his tone cut through my foggy haze of sleep. "Raissa, get up now." He didn't mince words, so I jumped out of bed, and my adrenaline jolted me into action.

Abba was standing over your crib. I joined him to check on you. To my horror, I looked down and your PEG had fallen out. The PEG is a small plastic feeding tube; it has an inflatable balloon on one end and a small cap on the other that opens for feeding. The balloon had burst, and the PEG had slid its way out of your body as if your body knew it didn't belong and was expelling it outward.

I went from adrenaline straight to panic. You were doing short breaks of twenty minutes at a time, and once we hit the twenty-minute mark, your sugars would drop, and we would have no way of feeding you. Abba called the emergency room and said to expect our arrival. I tried, without avail, to insert a new PEG where the old one had been. The nurses had walked me through the steps before, but I had never done it on my own—and certainly not under duress. I tried to insert the PEG into the gaping hole in your stomach. I had no time to be a mother right now. I was a nurse, and I banished my emotions to the deepest recesses of my mind and tried to focus on the task at hand. I couldn't even insert the new tube into the hole; it would not fit. I tried again. You were screaming. I am sure it was painful. I grabbed Vaseline (which I later found out should not be used, but I was desperate for time and out of options). I coated the tube in Vaseline and tried to insert it again but to no avail. Out of options and out of time. We gave you a glucagon injection that would maintain your sugars until we got to the hospital. We grabbed all your equipment and medications and sped to the hospital. In the pitch black, on an empty road, on the way to the emergency room. Again. Never a dull moment in this family.

In fact, I longed for dull moments. The boring and banal moments of life. I was tired of the constant state of crisis we found ourselves in. The never-ending marathon. The stress, the panic, the pressure to be good parents, good doctors, good nurses all at the same time. And, as it often did, the feeling of being overwhelmed overcame me, and I lost myself in despair.

This incident—and many others like it—reminded me of the fragility of our existence. Our lives, our mobility, our ability to exist as a family outside these hospital walls all depended on a little piece of plastic. Made in China. And it was terrifying.

CHAPTER 15

Parenthood

ONCE A FRIEND SENT ME an online quiz: "What kind of parent are you?" I clicked on the link, answering as honestly as I could, and as I finished and clicked the submit button. My answer popped up.

"Based on your answers you are an 'Overwhelmed Parent.'" The description continued on: "Every shower seems to you like a vacation." Ha! So true and so accurate.

Sometimes it feels like there is a line called *impossible*, and right above that is parenthood. So hard, so draining, and so rewarding at the same time. It's the hardest job I have ever loved, but it might just be killing me.

CHAPTER 16

Sesame Incident

ONE MORNING WE PACKED UP and went out to breakfast. Just your regular family (with your pump, continuous glucose monitor, and Joey pump, with continuous food through your PEG). But you wouldn't know it by looking at us. All covertly placed and discreetly hidden. Just your regular first-time parents out with their infant.

You were sleeping in your stroller, so like any other parents, we took the time to leisurely order, sip our coffee, and soak up a few moments of peace and quiet. You woke up just as breakfast arrived. Murphy's Law of parenthood—just as you sit down to eat a nice meal or to curl up with a hot cup of coffee to enjoy a moment to yourself, the baby wakes up. Every time.

Just as breakfast arrived, you awoke. You were immediately restless. As we snacked on fresh baguettes, fruits, and cheese, I suggested to your abba that we give you a bite. You weren't yet eating with your mouth. That was another challenge that we weren't ready to face. There were too many other pressing issues. He scooped up a bite of *techina*, a Middle Eastern dip similar to hummus and made out of sesame.

As it turns out, sesame is the third-most-prevalent allergy of babies, right behind peanut butter and milk. You had an immediate reaction. First, you threw up. Projectile-vomit throwing up. Then your face started to swell.

It's a scary feeling when the fight-or-flight response takes over your body. I froze. I felt the fear grip me and numb me from the inside out. The tightness in my chest took over my limbs and mind. Everything froze. Complete numbness.

Thankfully, your abba was quicker on his feet. He paid the bill and exited quickly, looking for a cab to flag down to take us to the hospital. You continued to get worse, so he called the local emergency ambulatory services, Magen David Adom, known as one of the best and most responsive emergency services in the world. They came within minutes.

We transferred you quickly and carefully out of your stroller into the ambulance. You were still hooked up to your Joey. So I sat in the back of the ambulance with you on my lap, your CGM in one hand and your Joey in the other. The ambulance drove speedily down the road and stopped when it crossed paths with another ambulance. They transferred us from one ambulance to another. The second ambulance had an on-call physician who administered epinephrine on the spot.

Your face began to clear up, and the swelling subsided. The ambulance sped along to the hospital. By the time the ambulance pulled up to the hospital, you were completely fine. I was not. The stress of the episode, my paralysis, my powerlessness, combined with a rocky ambulance ride, turned my stomach, and as they took the gurney out of the ambulance to wheel you into the PICU, I fell out of the ambulance and blindly groped my way through the alley to find an appropriate spot to throw up.

I told Abba and the ambulance team that I would catch up with them. I just needed a few minutes to catch my breath and get some fresh air. Once I composed myself, I entered the PICU to find your bed. Fortunately, the first face I saw was a familiar one: Dr. House, a young, bright doctor whom we had aptly nicknamed for his creative, outside-the-box thinking and consistent stream of new theories and diagnoses during our time in the NICU. He gave me a big smile.

"Well, the good news is that you brought in a perfectly healthy child," he said, "aside from his underlying condition, of course."

We stayed for a few hours for observation, and then they released us. Let me tell you, I did not miss that place at all. No love lost.

And boy, did I punish myself. What a stupid mistake. What a stupid, preventable mistake. After everything we had already been through. I could have saved us a trip to the hospital.

I would never feel the same way about sesame again.

CHAPTER 17

Full Circle

I REMEMBER LAST YOM KIPPUR, the holy Jewish Day of Atonement. Ten days after you were born. Lying on the floor in our small, sterile hospital hostel room. Pounding my fists to the ground. Sobbing, begging, praying that I would get to keep you. You were up on the ninth floor in the NICU hooked up to a cocktail of medications and IVs. You were getting continuous food and assistance breathing with the oxygen tubing. Your monitors for heart rate, breathing rate, oxygen saturation, and blood pressure were constantly beeping, signifying that they were abnormal.

I remember being so angry. Why? Why us? Why my son? Why my family? Pounding the ground. Please leave us alone, let us be. Let this all be a bad dream. Let us go home and wake up in a completely different reality. Please don't let this be our reality. Pounding, pounding, sobbing. As if my tears could change the course of our future. As if my tears could transfer all your suffering to me.

I had lived a good life. A full life. A great childhood growing up in the deep woods of New Hampshire. I was very lucky. Excelled in school, achieved everything I set my mind to, had an amazing family and "ride or die" friends. I embarked on an adventure to move across the world to start a new life. I learned another language, another culture. I fell in love. I finished my second degree, an MBA in my second language. I was lucky enough to meet and marry the greatest man in the whole world.

I have already had a full life. Take me instead. Let him live. Take me instead.

I felt like my own version of Jean Valjean, my inner soul performing "Bring Him Home." But who was my audience? And so, I prayed, begged, pleaded with the God I no longer believed in. As Nietzsche wrote, "Not that you lied to me, but that I no longer believe in you, that is what has shaken me."

And here I am a year later. We've been home for months. You are down to only two medications! A huge accomplishment. Off continuous food, and we are down to very little medical equipment. Able to move freely about. And for that I am extremely grateful.

Every year, Yom Kippur is a time for reflection. Time for apologies. Time to make amends. And as I look back upon this year, I feel as though I didn't spend time with anyone but you. Certainly not enough time to warrant apologies. So I will begin my preparations for Yom Kippur with a list of my apologies to you. And I hope that you can find it in your heart to forgive me.

To my darling son,

I am sorry. I am sorry that I could not be the mother that I wanted to be. I am sorry that I could not protect you. I am sorry that you were given such a rough start to life, and I am so proud of everything you have overcome. You have been through more in your one year than most people go through in a lifetime, and I am sorry that I did not have the power to change the cards that you were dealt.

I am sorry that you did not get to enjoy being a baby, and I am sorry that I did not enjoy being a mother more. Now it is easy to enjoy your babbles, laughs, and the shadows you make on the wall. But in the beginning, we did not have the luxury of time. I am sorry that your health was so unstable, and I am grateful to be able to now see your trajectory toward recovery. It wasn't always that way. Either way I used to look, backward or forward, I used to just see despair and darkness. I am sorry I wasn't always optimistic, and I am sorry that I had moments of despair when I almost gave up. Those were my weakest moments, and I am not proud of them.

I am sorry that I was more of a nurse and a doctor and a data analyst than your mother those first few months. I am sorry that we were stuck in the hospital for all those months, and I am sorry that your entire world, our entire world, consisted of fluorescent lights, hospital monitors, and alarms. I wanted to introduce you to Bach and fresh air and sunlight and nature long before you were stable enough to experience it.

Most of all, I am sorry that I was so powerless. Our circumstances were so beyond my control. As a mother, as a parent, I only want the best for you, but sometimes circumstances are too gray to decipher what the best is. What I can say is that I tried, I know that I tried, advocated, and fought for you as hard as I could. But unfortunately in this life, trying, fighting—this effort is less than half the battle. So many things are beyond human control and need to be aligned in order for life to be smooth sailing. I am sorry that I used to take that for granted. I never will again.

I love you always. May you be sealed in the Book of Life and may your years only get better and easier. You deserve it.

Love,
Ima

CHAPTER 18

Fragility

In the end, I came to the conclusion that Yom Kippur is about the fragility of life.

But I don't need to be reminded of that. I know it all too well. I know how many millions and billions of things need to go right in order for you to produce a thought, a word. How your entire body protects the functioning of your brain. Your brain is the headquarters, and all the rest of the gladiators—your major organs, your minor organs, your heart, your lungs, kidneys, pancreas, stomach, your skin, your skeleton—all play a vital role. They all work really hard in order to protect and support brain function. And if just one fails, well, the lights go out, the offices close one by one in headquarters. When you faint, it happens slowly: your vision, and then your hearing, and one by one, the office lights go dark in headquarters.

Well, I wish that you should never know. We are lucky so far in that your sugars have never been low enough, for long enough, for you to lose consciousness, to collapse into a seizure, to suffer permanent brain damage. But many hyperinsulinemia patients do, and it's not an uncommon phenomenon.

This whole time, we have been working so hard, been so diligent, so vigilant, because we know that if we slip, if we relax, if we lose track of time, there is always a risk at headquarters. And that is a huge burden to bear. Sometimes my shoulders collapse under the responsibility, and sometimes it just seems too big a load for a parent to carry.

So I do not need a special day reminding me how precious life is. How special it is. How fragile it is. How difficult it is to come into being. And to be. Year after year.

I know that each day is a blessing. Even when it feels like a curse.

CHAPTER 19

The Joy of Motherhood

And then there are the good days. The ones when I just get to be a mother. The ones when your sugars are stable and we get to play and focus more on your development and less on your health.

So Saba and Safta bought you a wagon—a beautiful red wagon—and you've been pushing it around the house, with parental supervision, for days. Slowly, cautiously learning to take steps. Learning control. Abba and I follow you around, stabilizing the wagon as you push. And this morning...*bam!* You woke up. Stood up and off you went. All by yourself. You were practically running around the house pushing your wagon. You were so proud of yourself.

And I was so proud of you; that moment felt so good. We've had so many dark times, so many struggles, so many obstacles to overcome that we must celebrate all the small—but hard-won—victories. And this was such a victory. Hooray for you!

CHAPTER 20

Victory

You remember the terrible, horrible, no good, very bad day? Well, today was the exact opposite of that.

It started with our regular hospital visit to Dr. Smith. We had tried to move you to Sandostatin one last time, and we were concerned about your liver function. Your last blood check was borderline above normal, but your numbers had dropped and were perfectly fine this time. Abba and I breathed a huge sigh of relief upon hearing this, because the Sandostatin had been our Hail Mary. We were loath to go back to the glucagon after a few quieter, more stable months thanks to the Sandostatin. This was also the third time we'd tried Sandostatin—once when we were in the NICU and another time as a trial off the glucagon, but both times it had negatively affected your liver. I was not excited—I was even discouraged—to try it a third time, but Dr. Smith made a very bold, calculated move and encouraged us to try one last time. This time we started at the lowest dosage possible in conjunction with the glucagon pump and slowly transitioned you away from the glucagon to the Sandostatin, and then we slowly tapered off the glucagon. And *ta-da!*

The Sandostatin is the Zeus of all gods. The most potent and powerful, and all other medications seem like nothing in its presence.

Also, we switched your PEG to a cute little gastrostomy button. It's much more manageable and less obtrusive, and it marks the occasion of you switching off continuous food to intermittent bolus feeding. Another huge triumph! We are so proud of you.

Lastly, during our meeting today, Dr. Smith said that given the look of things, he believes that you are going into remission. *Remission.* I went spontaneously deaf when I heard that and asked him to repeat himself a few times. He said that you are on a low-enough dosage that it looks like you are going into remission.

It has been one hell of a year for us. One hell of a lifetime for you. And, please God, things are looking up from here on out. Dr. Smith said to us, in a very fatherly manner, that he was very proud of you and of us as a family and how we've handled everything. It meant a lot, since this year has been nothing short of impossible. And his acknowledgment of our hard work made us feel proud of the work we have done as parents.

I am so proud of you, my little fighter, for all you have been through, for all you have overcome. For who you are and how you've handled everything. I wish for you that the worst is behind us. I wish for you all the world has to offer you and that it only gets better and better with time. You have been in hospitals for more than your fair share, and, whether or not you remember, you've seen and witnessed more horrors than most. I wish that from here on out, you will get to see and experience only the beauty, glory, and joy that life has to offer.

We are so proud of you, our little boy.

CHAPTER 21

Another Victory

When I was in high school, as one of the only Jews at a predominantly Waspy boarding school, I was selected to attend a conference on diversity in private schools. I was one of the only white participants in attendance.

We did a number of interesting "getting to know the participants" games, and I remember one of them very vividly. All the conference participants were asked to stand in a long horizontal line, facing the same way, in a large auditorium. We were asked to close our eyes and were then asked a series of questions: some geographical, some socioeconomic, and some personal. If the answer was yes, you took a step forward. If it was no, you took a step back.

"Did you have hot meals and enough food in your house growing up?"

"Did your parents tell you they love you?"

At the end of the series of questions, we were told to open our eyes and look around. I was very close to the wall, but there were others closer and others very far behind. We were told that on three, we were to run to the wall, and whoever arrived first won.

Now, I don't remember whether the winner actually won anything, but it was a really memorable lesson in the facts of life. Some are privileged and start out ahead, and others, while they can run as hard as they can, will never catch up. I noticed then how privileged I was among this bunch and how many opportunities I had been given that put me "ahead."

I thought of this game, which I played almost fifteen years ago, on Monday, when I took you to your first music class, our first mommy-baby extracurricular activity. You loved class—seeing the other kids, playing with the instruments. You were even trying to sing along. It was so adorable.

And as I looked around the music circle, it occurred to me that this was a big milestone. You worked so hard to get here. Harder than any other kid sitting around that circle. I had probably worked harder than any other mommy to get you there.

Every class, every outing, every trip to the playground was a victory. We felt the sun shine brighter, we felt the fresh air in our lungs and on our skin, and we enjoyed every moment together, as we would never again take our mobility for granted.

We still have a ways to go. But the victories must be celebrated, and this was certainly one of them.

Part III

CHAPTER 1

Returning to Work

My maternity leave felt like an eternity. I would have killed to just be another mom trying to juggle work and home life. When I was seven, I told my mother, a pulmonologist and adult intensive care specialist, that when I grew up, I was going to be an artist so that I could actually spend time with my children. I actually don't remember that story, but she'll never forget it.

I wanted normalcy—I wanted my regular, boring life back. So as I geared up to return to work, I wanted to acknowledge all the support that my company, let's call them *Hattan*, had provided during our challenging time. So I wrote the following letter. I wasn't sure to whom I should address it, so I wrote it to the CEO and all of the vice presidents of human resources. It went something like this:

June 15, 2014

Dear CEO and management team,

I am writing this letter to thank the entire Hattan family for all you have done for us. As I am gearing up to rejoin the working Hattan community from maternity leave, I would feel remiss if

I didn't formally thank the team and all the Hattan resources available to us during what has been the most difficult time in my life.

First, I would like to introduce myself, and then I will share with you the highlights of this past year and the ways in which Hattan supported us during this significant and transformative journey into parenthood.

My name is Raissa Hacohen, and I was born in Nashua, New Hampshire. I attended the Groton School and Brown University and then ended up moving abroad to Israel to complete my MBA at Hebrew University. I met and married my husband in Jerusalem, and in September 2013, I was a healthy, pregnant twenty-nine-year-old poised to enter motherhood.

Everything changed as our son was born. I was rushed to the hospital for an emergency C-section, and after significant testing, my son was diagnosed with hyperinsulinemia, a childhood disease affecting his blood-sugar levels. As my son was admitted to the NICU, my husband and I never left his side. We moved into a small hostel inside of the hospital and remained there for four and a half months as we began to nurse him to health.

Having recently been onboarded, I took advantage of all of the Hattan resources available to my family. Firstly, I contacted the manager of the Expert Medical Opinion Program, who analyzed my son's charts, reached out to world-renowned specialists in the field, and provided critical feedback for his treatment. Secondly, my colleagues contacted the family emergency fund, and Hattan funded our entire hostel stay so that we could be vigilantly by his side. Thirdly, HR colleagues reminded us that there was an option of therapy sessions, also subsidized by Hattan, which we took advantage of to help get us through this difficult time. In addition, I received many visitors, supportive e-mails, and phone calls from Hattan colleagues across the globe.

My son is almost ten months old now and is doing so much better (almost unrecognizable compared to the newborn I held in my arms at the hospital). You can see his photo attached. As I gear up to return to work, I wonder how I can ever express my gratitude toward my colleagues and the company at large for the amazing resources it provided to my family. We thank you from the bottom of our hearts, and I look forward to rejoining and to contributing to the Hattan family.

Gratefully yours,
Raissa Hacohen

Surprisingly enough, I received a reply from the CEO's secretary that said he was away on business and would get back to me in a day or two. She also mentioned how cute you are in that photo.

Sure enough, two days later, I received a reply. Impressive from a CEO for a ninety-thousand-person company. It read something like this:

Raissa—first let me say that I am very pleased that your son is doing so well, and so are you and your husband.

Thank you for sending us your e-mail and sharing with us the sometimes-painful journey that your family has been on. I am so thankful and proud that the Hattan family and all of our resources were made available to you and your son to get you to a good place.

We are glad to have you rejoin the team, and your contributions to Hattan are all the gratitude you need to show us.

—CEO

Four months after I returned from maternity leave, as part of its annual layoffs, Hattan cut 8 percent of its global workforce—six thousand jobs in total, and three hundred in the Jerusalem office, including mine.

So, I wrote again to the CEO.

Dear CEO,

I am writing to thank you again and give you an update on my son's situation.

I was in touch when I returned to Hattan from maternity leave four months ago, and my son is now fourteen months and doing much better. You can see his photo attached. He is the sweetest little boy, and you would never know all that he has dealt with and overcome in his short lifetime.

I am writing you a final thank-you. I was recently part of the 8 percent of the Hattan workforce in the LR. Hattan was wonderfully supportive to us during the most difficult time in our lives, and I was truly looking forward to dedicating my career to repaying the large debt that I owe this company.

With warm regards,
Raissa

Raissa—I am both glad that Hattan could be there for you and your family during the difficult times and saddened to know that you were part of the LR. Regrettably, the company had to make some pretty difficult decisions that affected many good employees.

Please send me pictures from time to time of your son as he continues to grow.

Sincerely,
CEO

Terribly disappointing. I was taught that with great power comes great responsibility. Too bad corporate America didn't learn the same.

CHAPTER 2

A Job Lost and Found

My boss—let's call him Ned—who was in Atlanta, scheduled a phone call with me on Sunday morning, 9:00 a.m. my time. That was my first red flag. Ned doesn't work on the weekends; he is a strict-office-hours kind of Peter Principle manager. And he definitely doesn't work at 2:00 a.m. on a Sunday his time.

Up to that point, I had heard about the expected layoffs, but my boss and boss's boss had assured me that our team had nothing to worry about. In addition, Israeli law protects mothers and ensures their job for three months after they return to the workplace. I was in month four, and after everything we'd already been through personally and all Hattan had invested in us, the possibility of being let go hadn't crossed my mind until I received Ned's invite.

Once I accepted his Outlook invitation, I knew it was the beginning of the end. Little did I know that it was also the beginning of a new beginning. I e-mailed Ned that I knew 9:00 a.m. was an ungodly hour on his end, that I was up from 6:00 a.m., and that he should feel free to call me late his time on Saturday evening.

The phone rang. I answered.

"Hi, Raissa. This is Ned."

"Hi, Ned."

"Well, Raissa, I hate to do this…but…" he began to stutter.

"Ned," I interrupted, "let's make this quick and painless, shall we?"

My assertiveness caught him off guard.

"Well, OK, Raissa, I have to read through this official document about the restructuring."

Hattan had internally given the "limited restructuring" the secret code name "Project Skyline," so anyone involved would know and anyone outside would think it was another customer project. "As you know," he began, "in August, Hattan announced a limited restructuring of eight percent of the Hattan workforce." As he read on, his voice faded into the background. My mind began to wander as I heard random groups of words: "limited restructuring…impacted our group…you are on notice…your position has been selected for elimination…you will have a hearing…share your thoughts…before a final decision is made."

Unbelievable, I thought. How could they do this to me? After all we've been through. This is the last thing I need. They had earned so much loyalty from me during my maternity leave, and I get fired five minutes later. Aside from the fact that I am a highly motivated, ambitious, and qualified employee with an Ivy League education and an international MBA, I could run our department better than 90 percent of the Hattan robots like Ned.

Fortunately, in Israel companies are required to go through a formal HR process before employees are fired. They scheduled a date for my hearing, and I came prepared to present my case.

Two weeks later I was called into a formal meeting with a Hattan manager and HR representative. She began with the same official speech: "As you know, in August, Hattan announced a limited restructuring of eight percent of the Hattan workforce..." She read the document in its entirety, even though I had heard it once. "Now is your opportunity to express anything you'd like to share."

I began by reading my initial letter to the company's CEO that I'd written before I returned from maternity leave, as well as his reply. I knew that many of the people being laid off were extremely qualified, so that strategy wouldn't work, but if I could play on the hierarchy that corporations worship so well, maybe I had a chance. I read the CEO's reply: "Thank you for sending us your e-mail and sharing with us the sometimes-painful journey that your family has been on. I am so thankful and proud that the Hattan family and all of our resources were made available to you and your son to get you to a good place. We are glad to have you rejoin the team, and your contributions to Hattan are all the gratitude you need to show us."

My voice quivered. "That was a short four months ago," I said. "And in this time, while I have accomplished many tasks and initiated projects, it is hardly the time needed to repay the great debt of gratitude that I owe this company."

And then I lost it completely. The manager ran out to get me a glass of water, and there was already a box of tissues strategically placed on the table. "In addition to returning from maternity leave, I still need to somehow provide my son with continuous care. We have monthly checkups at the hospital with his endocrinologist. My husband or I am with him all the time. We are also currently undergoing genetic mapping to evaluate whether this situation is preventable in the future. I hope that you will take all of these matters under consideration as you review my file." Not as composed as I would have liked, but I covered all of my prepared points.

"Thank you for your time," said the woman from HR. "Someone from the team will be in touch with you shortly."

I had heard that Hattan was giving out an additional five-month severance to all those fired. Other colleagues had received their official notices a day or two later. So when I was invited back into HR for another meeting the following week, I wasn't sure what to expect.

The same HR woman and her exact doppelganger were sitting around a round conference table. Both plain, heavyset, blond, and dispassionate. Dulled by years of sitting behind a desk pushing paper and other mindless, bureaucratic tasks, which I normally call "monkey work." So average and unmemorable that if you had a three-hour meeting with them face-to-face that wasn't about your future, you'd never remember it.

Since I had already gotten in the habit of nicknaming, I'll call them Tweedledee and Tweedledum.

Tweedledee began our second meeting in the same way as our first. "As you know, in August, Hattan announced a limited restructuring of eight percent off the Hattan workforce…" She read the document in its entirety again. "Since you shared such a compelling story in our last meeting, Hattan would like to offer you a seven-month severance package. Regular Hattan employees are receiving one month's notice plus five months' severance, and Hattan would like to give you two months' notice plus a seven-month severance package."

"So I am fired?" I asked, confused. "But for more money?"

"Well," she continued, "your position has been selected for elimination. We would like to offer you this package, and if you accept you will be required to sign a mutual-separation agreement."

What is that? I thought to myself. Why would they offer me more money? Was Hattan being a benevolent dictator, or was I missing something? Corporations don't usually act out of selflessness, but they were good to me before; maybe this is a bittersweet good-bye? Is that possible?

"Why don't you take a day to think about it, and then we'll meet to sign the paperwork," she suggested.

And just like that, the meeting was over, and I was left wondering what had just happened. Did I just get fired for a second time? Why would they offer me more money to leave? I went to my office and shut the door. My head fell into my lap. I was so angry and confused. Hadn't I been through enough? I was so angry for being fired, and for some reason, offering me more money only added insult to injury.

In my first two HR meetings, I had felt disempowered. Unfamiliar with the process and unsure of myself since my return from maternity leave, I had been a passenger on the Hattan train to unemployment. But for my third meeting, I came fully prepared, guns blazing. I had done my homework this time. As I suspected, Hattan was not a benevolent dictator, and, after a brief consultation with my lawyer friend, I realized that Israeli law protects women across a variety of medical categories. Apparently, our genetic-mapping process with the hospital technically fell into a gray area under one of these categories, and as such I was legally protected. Hattan couldn't fire me without going through an extensive governmental legal process. This legal protection necessitated a mutual-separation agreement for Hattan to fire me. My lawyer friend assured me that if they could have legally fired me, they would have done it already. They couldn't hang me, but they could persuade me to hang myself. And such was the task of Tweedledee and Tweedledum.

With that knowledge and protection, I took my seat at the HR conference table for the third time with Tweedledee and Tweedledum. I had a clear strategy. This was a chess game, and if I played it correctly, I could keep my job. I angled my iPhone at the center of the table to record the conversation, should I need evidence for later.

Tweedledee repeated herself for the hundredth time: "As you know, in August, Hattan announced a limited restructuring of eight percent off the Hattan workforce...Hattan is offering a seven-month severance package, and to receive this package you will need to sign this agreement." She pushed the mutual-separation agreement across the table and handed me a pen.

I leafed through the paperwork and placed it back down on the table.

"Thank you for this generous offer," I said. "I certainly appreciate your efforts. Having said that, I am a highly qualified employee. I have an international MBA and an Ivy League undergraduate education. I am a hard worker, extremely dedicated to the success of this organization. I can provide references from my colleagues regarding my qualifications and contributions to this company. Given that, I would like to keep my job. If that is not possible, I would elect to stay within Hattan."

"Wouldn't you prefer some time off to spend with your son?" asked Tweedledum.

"That is what my maternity leave was for. Now I am back and eager to contribute to the success of this company."

"Well, your position has been eliminated, and it's not that easy just to find you a new position. If you were an engineer or developer, it would be easier to do, but that's not possible for an analyst position," said Tweedledee.

"Well," I began, "as of yesterday, I noted one hundred and twenty-one open analyst positions across Hattan, sixty-nine of which allow for flexible or remote work. In the past few weeks, I have applied to fifty-seven of those positions, which I thought were relevant. Wouldn't it be possible to help me move to one of those positions?" I asked, maintaining my composure. I had made a decision tree of all the possible moves and counter-moves, questions and counter-questions, answers and counter-answers. Where I was unprepared before, I was overly prepared now.

"Furthermore," I continued, "if I were to consider your package, which I am not, but if I were, it's too risky financially."

"What do you mean?" said Tweedledum, "It's a very generous package for a Hattan employee."

"I agree," I said. "It's a great package for a regular Hattan employee. But for an employee who is four months back from maternity leave, it's risky, and for an employee four months back from maternity leave with a baby at home who requires special attention, it's definitely too risky. Say, for example, I took your package and then I was unemployed and I got pregnant again in the next few months. I would be pregnant for nine months, where no one would hire me, plus four months of state-paid maternity leave—that's seventeen months, almost two years I would be out of the workforce. Lost salary, lost pension, lost bonuses, lost promotions, plus it's harder to get hired after being out of the workforce for that long."

"You can get hired while you're pregnant!" Tweedledum interjected. "You don't even have to tell them until you start showing."

That was just too dumb to dignify with a response.

"Nonetheless, it's too risky. If the risk was substantially mitigated, I would consider the package, but I would really prefer to keep my job. Hattan has ninety thousand employees, six thousand in Israel. I am sure that I am qualified for something. Obviously, you need to run this up the totem pole," I said patronizingly. "I'll be in my office for the next couple of hours, or we can schedule another meeting later in the week."

Boom! I slid the papers back onto the table gracefully. Tweedledee and Tweedledum looked at me with their mouths open. I left the conference door open behind me. My shoes clicked the floor as I exited toward the elevator, and I felt so good in that moment. Checkmate.

Meeting four was with Tweedledee. Tweedledum was on vacation.

Tweedledee: "As you know, in August, Hattan announced a limited restructuring of eight percent off the Hattan workforce." Shoot me if I have to hear this spiel one more time. "We understand that you were unhappy with the original severance offer." She walked over to the whiteboard in the meeting room and began to draw a diagram. "The original offer was two months on the payroll with a seven-month severance package. Our current offer is ten months of severance. You can have it as three months on the payroll with a seven-month severance package or two months on payroll with eight months of severance. It's your choice."

My mom used to use this strategy on my sister and me. Would you like to brush your teeth before or after the bath? Would you like to do the dishes before or after TV time? She was creating the illusion of choice. Would you like a five-foot or six-foot rope to hang yourself with? Velvet or satin?

I politely declined. It would be a nice cushion, but I really had nothing to lose in the long term. I needed to keep my job, and if it was my legal right, I would choose to exercise it.

The next day, I received a letter notifying me that my position had been eliminated, but I was still a Hattan employee, and I would still report to my current manager. Tweedledee concluded the process with a sneer, saying that I should consider these past few weeks as a gift from Hattan. She literally used the word "gift," since Hattan had not required me to count these past few weeks as vacation days.

I wanted to punch her in the face—or at least give her the finger—on my way out. But I was still a Hattan employee and she was a colleague, so I mustered my most genuine fake smile, accepted the letter, and exited for the elevator. I had achieved my objective, but for some reason, victory didn't feel particularly sweet.

I tasted the sweetness of victory a few weeks later when I found, interviewed for, and won a new position within Hattan, far outside of my current group. The position was not only a promotion, but I also beat out other candidates across Europe, as this position was originally offered in Brussels, and they relocated the position to Jerusalem to accommodate my location. And just like that, the Hattan employment rollercoaster was over... or at least on pause. And at least for the present moment, I felt like the odds were in my favor.

CHAPTER 3

Uncertainty

LIFE IS SO GODDAMN UNPREDICTABLE. And cruel.

We build these walls. Social constructs, as my professor at Brown would say. Walls made of ideas. Walls that fortress society and allow it to run smoothly. I work, I'll get a paycheck. I follow traffic laws, I'll be safe. Metaphorical walls that make life feel predictable, but it is all just an illusion. An illusion of reality.

In ancient times, different societies believed in a different god for every uncertainty. A god for protection. A god for fruitful crops. A god for rain. A god for bounty. A god for love. Their lives were by far more unpredictable than those in modern society. Although if you go to any third-world country today, you can still taste what a world of uncertainty is like. You live for the present day, as no one can guarantee what tomorrow will bring. A tsunami. A flood. A famine. A war. And so you pray to all your gods to keep the frail walls of your home, of your society intact for one more day.

In modern times, civilization built seemingly strong walls as daily life became more predictable and certain. Simultaneously, society whittled down its belief system. It abandoned gods. As society embraced monotheism, there was a shift in understanding that, while specific uncertainties remain, if you follow the rules of society, things will generally work out in your favor. The American dream. Work hard. Achieve. Build. Acquire.

But every time you find yourself face-to-face with one of those remaining uncertainties—illness, love, conception, pregnancy, birth, raising children—you are reminded just how terrifying this world is. How all the walls we build crumble under the weight of uncertainty. Just one thing can randomly go wrong, someone can fall chronically ill, couples can struggle with fertility, pregnancies can miscarry, and all the walls come tumbling down.

We create the illusion that we are in control. When things come crashing down, we realize that none of it is actually in our hands.

The one god that's left cannot close the gap on uncertainty. It's funny that modern-day society calls natural disasters "an act of God." Aren't we just acknowledging that the only god that remains is the master of uncertainty?

The god of unpredictability. And she is a bitch, isn't she?

CHAPTER 4

Sweet Taste of Freedom

And then the holidays roll around again and you are reminded of how far you've come.

Last year, we rolled you, my dear son, in your bassinet to Passover Seder at your grandfather's. You were hooked up to a continuous glucagon pump and a continuous feed of a Nutramigen-formula concoction to keep your sugars up, and despite that, your sugars still dropped. They plummeted at a moment's notice with no warning.

And this year, we approached freedom anew. Without a continuous feed, on a Sandostatin pump with three-hour breaks in between, when your sugars fall, they float. Slowly enough for us to manage, and even at one and a half years, you are old enough to communicate, to give us a specific signal, to tell us that your sugars need attending to. Such a smart boy. My darling, we are so proud of you. Of how far you've come.

Every time I take you to the park and you laugh gleefully on the swings, I am reminded that there was a time that you were hooked up to so many lifesaving machines, that swings—that any independent movement—weren't even an option. That wasn't such a long time ago. As the sun beats down on us, I think that you and I enjoy the park more than anyone else there. We appreciate the sun, the wind, the outdoors, because we were stuck inside for so many months under the fluorescent lights. We appreciate the swings, the slide, the merry-go-round because once you were not mobile. Hospital-bound and then homebound for such a long time. A jail with invisible walls. A lifesaving one, but a jail just the same. And now we are free. You are dependent on things but in a way that is totally manageable and almost second nature to us now. We are mobile, we are happy, and you are growing like such a big, strong boy. Beyond any scenario that I could have envisioned just a year ago. As painful as the memory is, it is just that—a memory. The wounds will be forever emblazoned, but the scars have begun to heal. Our physical and emotional scars have begun to disappear, and we have begun to heal.

And sometimes I think back. I think back to when we were barely living, slowly dying. I think about others. Those who are enslaved by life. Enslaved by death. I remember that time—those times—when your body could feel like a prison. And I think of those people and hope. (I didn't dare hope back then. Hope was too dangerous.) And now, I hope for a time when we can all be free.

CHAPTER 5

Happy Second Birthday

To MY DARLING SON, ON your second birthday.

There are no words. No words to express, no words to illuminate the depth of my pride. The height of my joy. The intensity of my love for you. And how much I treasure being your mother.

We have been through so much. So much in these two short years. Time has flown by, but there were times when it inched by, day by day, hour by hour.

There is no bigger transition, no more drastic change than that of becoming a first-time parent. I have never felt so broken or so whole, so high from your accomplishments and so low from your pain. Life was never so bright or so dark before I entered parenthood.

You have overcome so much in your brief time in this world. For that I am so proud and so grateful.

We still have our daily struggles. But it is mostly a story of management. Sugar management. Managing our daily schedule and life around your sugars and your many medical appointments. And mostly we have it down to a science. We don't really know parenthood any other way. And while there were definitely highs and lows, it has gotten so much easier and so much better. We went from hospitalization to homebound. From homebound to mobile. Incredible progress for only two years.

As I look back, I remember the dark times, when time felt like it had completely stopped. Our life had been suspended for the foreseeable future. And I want to tell that new mother, who is in the darkest place imaginable, that it will get easier, it will get better. Change is the only constant, even if you can't always feel it.

Now, I wake up every day, relish your morning smile, and cherish our morning reading time before breakfast. How you finish the rhymes in your *Hop on Pop* book and skip to your favorite pages, laughing uncontrollably, protesting when Pat sits on the cactus. I treasure our trips to the park and pushing you on the swing, as you laugh and giggle with pleasure. Every day is a wonder and a treasure.

I cherish these times all the more because it is a life that I never could have imagined, a life I never could have pictured in those first few months when we were confined to the hospital. I never could have imagined then that it would be this good, full of this much joy. I never could have imagined this much light amid all that darkness.

I could go on to build a billion-dollar company or cure cancer, and you would still be the achievement of which I am most proud.

As we celebrate your second birthday, I wish for you that it only continues to get better. That you are given only the best of what this life has to offer. That your health continues to improve and that you experience a full recovery. May you be blessed with health, joy, love, and amazing adventures, and may you always know that your ima loves you.

Love Always,
Ima

Epilogue

WHEN THIS MEMOIR IS PUBLISHED, you will be two and a half years old. From its inception to its publishing, you have grown from a newborn in the NICU into a little boy, and anyone who hasn't read this memoir would never know the difference. They would see an adorable little boy who is obsessed with cars and construction, *Hop on Pop* and *Peppa Pig*, who counts to ten and bosses everyone around. They would mistake us for any other loving parents trying to juggle it all and chase around an active little boy in the midst of his terrible twos.

I have written about being grateful but words cannot do the emotion justice. When I speak to others about what we've been through, I liken the process of becoming a patient (or the caregiver of a patient) to the five stages of grief: denial, anger, bargaining, depression, and acceptance. However, during a health crisis, the stages ebb and flow into each other. They circle back around in different shades, and the acceptance part is more elusive, as the outcomes of diagnoses and treatments are less clear and less finite. As I read over my words, some of which I wrote more than two years ago, I can find all those stages and emotions embedded in the chapters in various forms.

I no longer recognize that writer, that mother, that darkness. I remember her but I don't know her anymore. As we slowly fought tooth and nail for our regular lives back, we tried to forget, to put the darkness behind us, and to not let it affect our future. Now, we have the luxury of allowing ourselves to dream and to hope. In the comfort of our own home with the worst behind us, we can paint a bright future. A future filled with adventures, a future bright beyond recognition. The future that I imagined for you in the beginning, when life was pregnant with possibilities.

I wish I could say that I learned something from the experience. I wish I could say that something positive came of our story. All I know is that love makes you capable of anything. Looking back at this memoir, I never would have thought that I had the strength to contend with any of these challenges. Love transforms you and gives you superhuman strength. It is humanity's only superpower.

Let love be the music that carries you. Continue to hope. Continue to love. Continue to get out of bed in the morning and put one foot in front of the other. Just doing that makes you a very brave person.

About the Author

Raissa was born in New Haven, CT and grew up in Hollis, New Hampshire. She graduated Brown University with a degree in Middle Eastern Studies and earned an MBA from the Hebrew University of Jerusalem.

She began her career in venture capital in Israel, and then moved to the hi-tech world. She is currently focusing on digital health and improving the patient experience.

She lives in Jerusalem with her husband and son.

www.ingramcontent.com/pod-product-compliance
Lightning Source LLC
Chambersburg PA
CBHW051922170526
45168CB00001B/501
9781518816246